T0342364

Cardiopulmonary Exercise Testing
and
Cardiovascular Health

Edited by

Karlman Wasserman, MD, PhD

Professor of Medicine, Emeritus
Division of Respiratory and
Critical Care Physiology and Medicine
Department of Medicine
Harbor-UCLA Medical Center
University of California, Los Angeles
Torrance, California

Futura Publishing Company, Inc.
Armonk, NY

Library of Congress Cataloging-in-Publication Data

Cardiopulmonary exercise testing and cardiovascular health / edited by
    Karlman Wasserman.
        p. cm.
    Includes bibliographical references and index.
    ISBN 0-87993-700-9 (alk. paper)
        1. Heart failure—Pathophysiology. 2. Exercise tests.
    3. Cardiopulmonary system. 4. Pulmonary gas exchange.
    I. Wasserman, Karlman.
        [DNLM: 1. Exercise Test. 2. Cardiovascular Diseases—diagnosis.
    3. Heart Failure, Congestive—physiopathology. 4. Lung Diseases—
    diagnosis. 5. Pulmonary Gas Exchange.   WG 141.5.F9 C2673 2002]
    RC669.9. C32 2002
    616.1'075—dc21

                                                        2001055632

Published by
Futura Publishing Company
135 Bedford Road
Armonk, NY 10504
www.futuraco.com

LC#: 2001055632
ISBN#: 0-87993-700-9

Contributors

Pier Guiseppe Agostoni, MD, PhD   Instituto de Cardiologia, Milan, Italy

Timothy A. Bauer, MS   Section of Vascular Medicine, University of Colorado Health Sciences Center, Denver, CO

Romualdo Belardinelli, MD, FESC   Lancisi Institute, Department of Cardiology, Ancona, Italy

Caroline Bergmeier, MD   Herzzentrum Ludwigshafen, Department of Cardiology, Ludwigshafen, Germany

Maurizio Bussotti, MD   Centro Cardiologico Monzino, Milan, Italy

Andrew J.S. Coats, MA, DM, FRACP, FRCP, FESC, FACC   Viscount Royston Professor of Cardiology, National Heart and Lung Institute, London, UK

Alain Cohen-Solal, MD, PhD   Department of Cardiology, Hospital Beaujon, Clichy, France

Perry M. Elliott, MD   Department of Cardiological Sciences, St. George's Hospital Medical School, University of London, London, UK

Pierre Vladimir Ennezat, MD   Department of Cardiology, Hospital Beaujon, Clichy, France

Long Tai Fu, MD   President, The Cardiovascular Institute, Tokyo, Japan

Anselm K. Gitt, MD   Herzzentrum Ludwigshafen, Department of Cardiology, Ludwigshafen, Germany

Marco Guazzi, MD, PhD, FACC   Co-director, Heart Failure Unit, Institute of Cardiology, University of Milan, Milan, Italy

Adrian Hall, MB, FANZCA   Division of Anesthesia and Intensive Care, Western Hospital, Melbourne, Australia

William R. Hiatt, MD   Professor of Medicine, Section of Vascular Medicine, University of Colorado Health Sciences Center, Denver, CO

Michiaki Hiroe, MD   Associate Professor, Tokyo Medical and Dental University, Tokyo, Japan

Haruki Itoh, MD   Director of Internal Medicine, The Cardiovascular Institute, Tokyo, Japan

Soraya Jones, PhD   Department of Physiology, St. George's Hospital Medical School, University of London, London, UK

Kazuzo Kato, MD   The Cardiovascular Institute, Tokyo, Japan

Makoto Kato, MD   Director of Cardiac Rehabilitation, The Cardiovascular Institute, Tokyo, Japan

Franz X. Kleber, MD, PhD   Direktor del Klinik für Innere Medizin, Unfal Krankenhaus Berlin, Berlin, Germany

Akira Koike, MD   Director, The Cardiovascular Institute, Tokyo, Japan

Tomoko Maeda, BS   Exercise Physiology Laboratory, The Cardiovascular Institute, Tokyo, Japan

Donna Mancini, MD   Columbia Presbyterian Medical Center, New York, NY

William J. McKenna, MD, DSc   Professor of Cardiology, Department of Cardiological Sciences, St. George's Hospital Medical School, University of London, London, UK

Jonathan Myers, PhD   Clinical Assistant Professor, Cardiology Division, Palo Alto VAHCS/Stanford University Medical Center, Palo Alto, CA

Koichi Okita, MD   Cardiovascular Medicine, Hokkaido University Graduate School of Medicine, Sopporo, Japan

Paul Older, MB, FRCA, FANZCA, FFICANZA   Director of Intensive Care Unit, Division of Anesthesia and Intensive Care, Western Hospital, Melbourne, Australia

Kazuto Omiya, MD   Lecturer, Cardiology, St. Mariana University School of Medicine, Kanagawa, Japan

Naohiko Osada, MD   Assistant Professor, Cardiology, St. Mariana University School of Medicine, Kanagawa, Japan

Ronald J. Oudiz, MD, FACC   Assistant Professor of Medicine, Division of Cardiology, Harbor-UCLA Medical Center, Torrance, CA

Jochen Senges, MD, FACC, FESC   Herzzentrum Ludwigshafen, Department of Cardiology, Ludwigshafen, Germany

Sanjay Sharma, MD   Department of Cardiological Sciences, St. George's Hospital Medical School, University of London, London, UK

Lynne Warner Stevenson, MD   Associate Professor of Medicine, Harvard Medical School; Director of Cardiomyopathy and Heart Failure Program, Brigham & Women's Hospital, Boston, MA

William W. Stringer, MD Associate Professor, Division of Respiratory and Critical Care Physiology and Medicine, Harbor-UCLA Medical Center, Torrance, CA

Xing-Guo Sun, MD Division of Respiratory and Critical Care Physiology and Medicine, Harbor-UCLA Medical Center, Torrance, CA

Jean-Yves Tabet, MD Department of Cardiology, Hospital Beaujon, Clichy, France

Akihiko Tajima, BS Chief, Exercise Physiology Laboratory, The Cardiovascular Institute, Tokyo, Japan

Maria Tokmakova, MD Department of Internal Medicine, Higher Medical Institute, Plovdiv, Bulgaria

Karlman Wasserman, MD, PhD Professor of Medicine, Division of Respiratory and Critical Care Physiology and Medicine, Harbor-UCLA Medical Center, Torrance, CA

Hiroshi Watanabe, MD The Cardiovascular Institute, Tokyo, Japan

Peer E. Waurick, MD Klinik für Innere Medizin, Unfal Krankenhaus Berlin, Berlin, Germany

Brian J. Whipp, PhD, DSc Professor of Physiology, Department of Physiology, St. George's Hospital Medical School, University of London, London, UK

Preface

This monograph describes new research and findings relevant to cardiovascular health as assessed by cardiopulmonary exercise testing (CPET). The primary role of the cardiovascular system is to supply O_2 to the metabolically active cells for the purpose of releasing energy from food substrate. O_2 is needed to oxidize food substrate for production of the chemical energy (high-energy phosphate) to support the energetic requirements of life, i.e., synthesis, active transport, and muscle contraction. Exercise is a special challenge to the cardiovascular system because the muscle energy requirement and therefore its O_2 requirement are greatly increased. For instance, to regenerate the energy to sustain walking at a pace of 3 miles per hour, the muscle O_2 requirement must increase approximately 20 times over that at rest. The ability of the cardiovascular system to speed up the supply of O_2 to sustain exercise is the most direct measure of cardiovascular health.

While the concept of evaluating a person's cardiovascular system by exercise testing is not new, the way it is done now is new. Computers and rapidly responding gas analyzers make it possible to evaluate the response of the cardiovascular system as a whole and its individual parts, including the heart, in a quantitative way. This contrasts with the way exercise stress tests are done in most clinical settings where only evidence for myocardial ischemia is investigated with electrocardiographic monitoring.

The contributors to this monograph are cardiologists and scientists who have a wealth of experience in CPET. The purpose of this book is to bring together these experiences in their use of CPET to quantify cardiovascular health and cardiovascular impairment of patients with a variety of cardiovascular illnesses.

The monograph is divided into four parts: 1) discussion of basic mechanisms involved in the regeneration of high-energy phosphate and effect on exercise gas exchange; 2) critical evaluation of various parameters of aerobic function and gas exchange efficiency, determined during CPET, to predict prognosis and survival time of patients with heart failure; 3) presentation of new research in the use of CPET to evaluate functional severity of coronary artery disease, pulmonary vascular disease, peripheral arterial disease, cardiac diastolic dysfunction, and the risk of a cardiovascular death following major surgery in the elderly; and 4) use of CPET to assess clinical course and effectiveness of therapy. Thus, this is a comprehensive presentation and an updating of what can be achieved to assess cardiovascular health with CPET. This is a new era in which the availability of reliable instrumentation and graphical presentation of function enable the physician and investigator to quantify the degree of success with which the cardiovascular system supports the energy-generating mechanisms needed to sustain life.

Karlman Wasserman, MD, PhD
Editor

Contents

Section 1

Physiological Basis of Cardiopulmonary Exercise Testing

1

Circulatory Coupling of External to Muscle Respiration During Exercise

Karlman Wasserman, MD, PhD,
William W. Stringer, MD, Xing-Guo Sun, MD, and
Akira Koike, MD

To perform exercise, chemical energy in the form of adenosine triphosphate (ATP) must be continuously regenerated in the muscles by mitochondrial respiration (O_2 consumption and CO_2 production). The major immediate role of the cardiovascular and ventilatory systems in response to exercise is to support muscle respiration. The ability of the cardiovascular and ventilatory systems to adequately support muscle respiration during exercise is a measure of their functional health.

Coupling of O_2 Uptake ($\dot{V}O_2$) to Work

Chemical energy in the form of high-energy phosphate bonds (~P) of ATP is transduced to mechanical energy for muscle contraction.[1] The regeneration of ~P can come from three mechanisms. The first and most important is that generated by muscle bioenergetic mechanisms involving molecular O_2 in mitochondria (Fig. 1). The mitochondria are the major site of ATP production. The two other sources of ATP are anaerobic mechanisms. The magnitude of $\dot{V}O_2$ at the lung in response to exercise depends on the work rate. The kinetics of $\dot{V}O_2$ depend largely on how adequately the circulation couples external respiration to muscle respiration (Fig. 1). The size of the contribution of the two anaerobic sources for regenerating ATP, splitting

From Wasserman K (ed): *Cardiopulmonary Exercise Testing and Cardiovascular Health.* Armonk, NY: Futura Publishing Company, Inc.; © 2002.

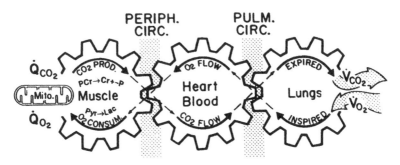

Figure 1. Circulatory coupling of muscle to external respiration. The gears connote that the circulation couples ventilation and gas exchange at the airway to muscle respiration. The muscle regenerates high-energy phosphate bonds by aerobic metabolism in the form of adenosine triphosphate (ATP) in the mitochondria (illustrated in the muscle gear). ATP can also be regenerated anaerobically by splitting phosphocreatine (PCr) and anaerobic glycolysis (Pyr→Lac) (see muscle gear). The first mechanism causes $\dot{V}O_2$ and $\dot{V}CO_2$ to increase in proportion to work rate in a ratio dependent on the metabolic substrate. The second and third mechanisms are anaerobic and therefore do not directly affect $\dot{V}O_2$ but do determine CO_2 output, the former lowering CO_2 output and the latter increasing it. See text for details. Modified from reference 17.

of phosphocreatine (PCr) and anaerobic glycolysis, also depends on how effectively the circulation couples external respiration to cellular respiration. The two anaerobic mechanisms of ATP regeneration operate only transiently during exercise and need to be restored by aerobic (O_2-requiring) mechanisms in recovery. These mechanisms account for a major part of the O_2 debt.

Of the two anaerobic sources of ~P that contribute to exercise bioenergetics (Fig. 1), the first in time sequence is that derived from the hydrolysis of intramuscular PCr.[2] Because the circulation cannot respond as quickly as muscle contraction can be initiated, muscle PCr serves as a reserve source of ~P to regenerate muscle ATP at the myofibril. This source of ~P is immediately available at the start of exercise to supplement the ATP in the muscle. Its contribution is complete by the time $\dot{V}O_2$ reaches a steady state.[3,4]

When PCr is split, the cellular pH turns alkaline because PCr, an acid molecule at cellular pH, produces neutral creatine and a mix of dibasic and monobasic phosphate with a pK (6.8) close to the pH of the cell.[5,6] The resulting alkalization of the cell causes cation (K^+) excess in the cell and a deficit of H^+.[7] Thus, CO_2, hydrated to H_2CO_3, dissociates into HCO_3^- and H^+. The alkaline cell takes up the latter while the former serves to balance the positive charge of K^+ liberated by the decrease in negative charges in the myocyte when PCr undergoes hydrolysis (Fig. 2). The net effect of this reaction is the fixation of metabolic CO_2 as HCO_3^- during this early period of exercise. The increase in HCO_3^- balancing the K^+, as it leaves

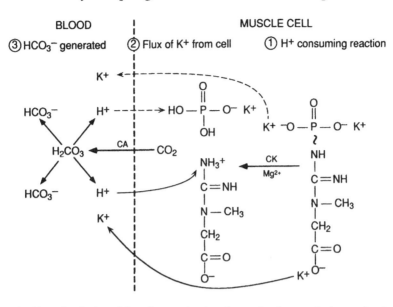

Figure 2. Hypothesis describing the mechanism for early changes in femoral vein pH, HCO_3^-, and K^+ in response to exercise. *Step 1* shows that when phosphocreatine (PCr) is hydrolyzed into creatine and inorganic phosphate, H^+ is consumed resulting in a reduction of negative charges in the cell and an alkalinizing reaction. *Step 2* illustrates that the excess in intracellular cation and a shortage of H^+ causes K^+ to leave the cell and H^+ to enter the cell. *Step 3* shows that the resulting efflux of K^+ from the cell is balanced by newly formed HCO_3^- in the fluid around the cell and effluent blood. Thus, metabolic CO_2, when hydrated, becomes H_2CO_2, which dissociates into H^+, which is taken up by the alkaline myocyte and HCO_3^- anion, which serves to balance the positive charge of K^+. From Wasserman et al.[7] with permission.

the myocyte, is reflected in the venous blood draining from the exercising muscle.[7] Thus, femoral vein pH, HCO_3^-, and K^+ increase concurrently (Fig 3). PCO_2 does not increase during this early period of exercise, despite an increase in $\dot{V}O_2$ and decrease in O_2 partial pressure (PO_2), because metabolic CO_2 is being rapidly fixed as HCO_3^- (Fig. 3). As a result, the respiratory exchange ratio (RER) decreases during this early period of exercise (Figs. 3 and 4). Chuang et al.[8] pointed out that about two thirds of the metabolic CO_2 retained in the body, accounting for the slow increase in CO_2 production ($\dot{V}CO_2$) relative to $\dot{V}O_2$ and the decrease in RER during the first 3 minutes of exercise (Fig. 4), was attributable to PCr hydrolysis. The remainder is attributable to the increase in CO_2 dissolved in tissues as tissue PCO_2 increases and to the increase in CO_2 in venous blood due to the Haldane effect (increased binding of CO_2 due to decreasing venous oxyhemoglobin saturation). The increase in CO_2 content in venous blood, other than that due to the Haldane effect, is not part of this component because it is closely offset by the unmeasured O_2 consumed from the venous blood during the same period of exercise.

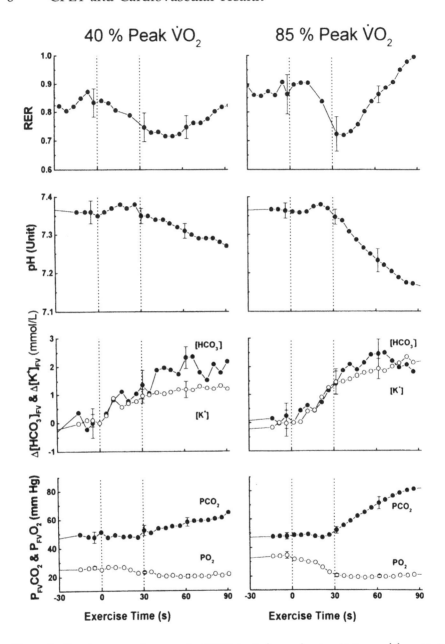

Figure 3. Respiratory exchange ratio ([RER] top), femoral vein pH (second from top), change (Δ) in femoral vein HCO_3^- and K^+ concentration (third from the top), and femoral vein PCO_2 and PO_2 in response to the start of exercise (zero time) for the first 90 seconds of upright leg cycling exercise at 40% (left panels) and 85% (right panels) of $\dot{V}O_2$peak. Each point is average of 5 subjects. Vertical bars on select points are SE values. Modified from Wasserman et al.[7]

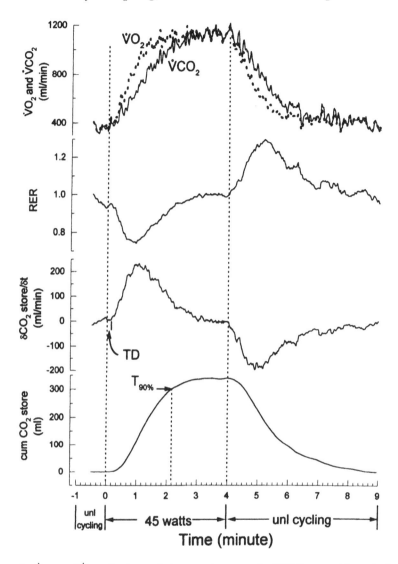

Figure 4. $\dot{V}_{O_2}$ and $\dot{V}_{CO_2}$ (top), respiratory exchange ratio ([RER] second from top), rate of change in CO_2 (third from top), and the cumulative change in CO_2 store (bottom) in response to a 4-minute 60-W constant work rate upright leg cycling exercise, starting at zero time, and 5-minute unloaded cycling recovery period. The data are second-by-second averages of 4 replicate tests. From Chuang et al.[8]

The second anaerobic mechanism, the anaerobic degradation of glycogen or glucose to lactate, starts after 30 seconds of exercise if the circulatory delivery of O_2 is inadequate.[7] This source of ATP is particularly important when the energy requirement exceeds the sum of PCr splitting and the aerobic regeneration of ~P,[9-12] e.g., when the cytoplasmic redox state decreases. This is an exercise intensity defined as being above the subject's anaerobic threshold (*AT*) (pathway B in Fig. 5).[12,13] Because O_2 transport is cardiovascular system dependent, the *AT* should be a particularly important measure of the level of work that can be sustained aerobically, i.e., without invoking anaerobic glycolysis (lactic acidosis).[14]

Effect of Anaerobic Source of ~P on Muscle Venous PCO_2 and HCO_3^- During Exercise

In the steady state of exercise, all of the energy required to support exercise is generated by aerobic mechanisms involving mitochondria. In this state, glycolysis is aerobic (Fig. 5, pathway A) and the rate of regeneration of ~P bonds can be calculated from the O_2 consumption. The two anaerobic mechanisms, while not requiring O_2 during exercise, affect HCO_3^- and PCO_2 in the femoral vein blood during leg cycling exercise in opposite ways and cannot be predicted from the changes in femoral vein PO_2 (Fig. 6). Because the splitting of PCr alkalinizes the muscle and the blood flowing through it, with the formation of HCO_3^- from metabolic CO_2, HCO_3^- initially increases in the femoral venous blood without an increase in femoral venous PCO_2 (Fig. 3). PCO_2 does not increase in the femoral vein during this early period of exercise despite a decrease in femoral vein PO_2 (Figs. 3 and 6). During exercise of heavy intensity, after femoral vein PO_2 stops decreasing, femoral vein HCO_3^- decreases and PCO_2 increases as HCO_3^- buffers the newly formed lactic acid (Fig. 6).

Muscle-Capillary Gas Exchange and the Critical Capillary PO_2

Figure 7 is a model of the microcirculation-muscle unit describing the pattern of fall in capillary PO_2 from the arterial to venous side of the capillary bed. The capillary PO_2 depends on the relationship between the O_2 flow to the O_2 consumption of the muscle ($\dot{Q}m \times O_2$ content/$\dot{V}O_2m$). The O_2 flow to muscle ($\dot{Q}m \times O_2$ content) must obviously exceed the muscle O_2 consumption ($\dot{V}O_2m$) to provide a capillary PO_2 driving pressure sufficient to avoid lactic acidosis resulting from anaerobic glycolysis. The minimal driving pressure needed to prevent muscle anoxia and anaerobic glycolysis is the critical capillary PO_2 (ccPO_2).[15] The muscle is never completely anoxic because the PO_2 is high on the arterial end of the capillary, i.e., above the ccPO_2. Anaerobic glycolysis, with net increase in lactate production, must develop in the myocyte where the capillary PO_2 reaches the ccPO_2, i.e., toward the venous end of the capillary.

Isolated mitochondria can respire and rephosphorylate adenosine diphosphate to ATP at a PO_2 of 1 mm Hg or less[16]; however, to sustain muscle mitochondrial respiration during exercise, the capillary PO_2 must be

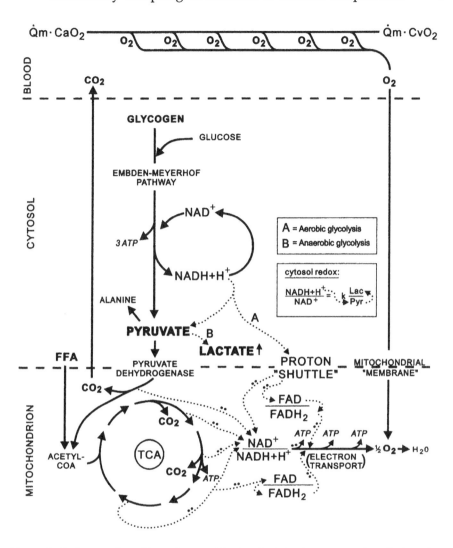

Figure 5. Pathways of aerobic and anaerobic glycolysis for the regeneration of adenosine triphosphate (ATP) in response to exercise. As long as O_2 flow through the muscle is sufficient to provide a driving pressure for O_2 to maintain adequate aerobic regeneration of ATP in the mitochondria to satisfy the muscle ATP need, cytosolic NADH + H^+ will be reoxidized by the mitochondrial membrane shuttle (pathway A). When the O_2 flow is insufficient to keep the mitochondrial membrane shuttle reoxidized, NADH + H^+ will be reoxidized back to NAD^+ by pathway B. This will result in an increase in cell lactate in proportion to the increase in cytosolic NADH + H^+/NAD^+ ratio (lowering of redox state). Qm = muscle blood flow; CaO_2 = arterial O_2 content; CvO_2 = muscle venous O_2 content; TCA = tricarboxylic acid cycle. Modified from Wasserman.[17]

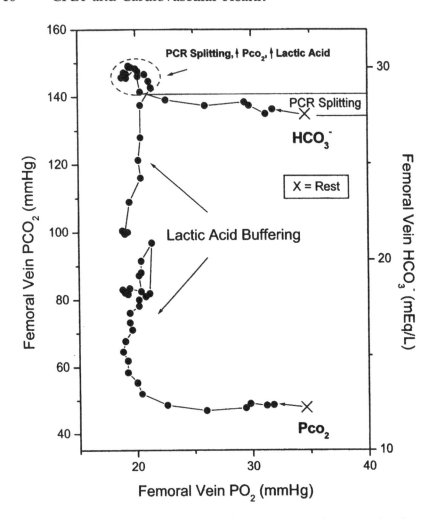

Figure 6. Change in femoral vein PCO_2 and HCO_3^- as PO_2 decreases after the start of heavy (85% of $\dot{V}O_2$max) exercise. The direction of change is from the resting value (X), leftward. Each subsequent point leftward is recorded from femoral vein blood sampled at 5-second intervals. The increase in femoral vein HCO_3^- during the first 30 seconds occurs without an increase in PCO_2. Thus, this is a true metabolic alkalosis resulting from the hydrolysis of phosphocreatine (PCR) as described in Fig. 2. Lactic acid production starts after the minimal (critical) capillary PO_2 is reached. Thus, femoral vein HCO_3^- decreases and PCO_2 increases due to the buffering of lactic acid in the exercising muscle, without a further fall in femoral vein PO_2. The data are the average of 5 normal subjects taken from Stringer et al.[18]

appreciably greater than 1 mm Hg for O_2 to diffuse from the red cell to the sarcoplasm. Wittenberg and Wittenberg[15] estimated that the "critical" capillary PO_2 driving pressure was between 15 and 20 mm Hg. Failure for O_2 flow to keep pace with the metabolic demand will cause the capillary blood PO_2 to reach its critical level before it exits the muscle-capillary func-

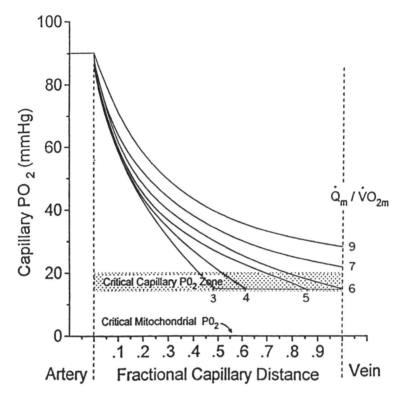

Figure 7. Model of muscle-capillary O_2 partial pressure (PO_2) as blood travels from artery to vein. The model assumes hemoglobin concentration of 15 g/dL, arterial PO_2 of 90 mm Hg, a mitochondrial PO_2 of about 1, and a linear O_2 consumption along the capillary. The rate of fall of capillary PO_2 must depend on the muscle blood flow ($\dot{Q}m$)/muscle $\dot{V}O_2$ ($\dot{V}O_2m$) ratio. The curves include a Bohr effect due to a respiratory CO_2 production. The end-capillary PO_2 cannot decrease below the critical capillary PO_2. The critical capillary PO_2 zone is taken from the work of Wittenberg and Wittenberg[15] Any muscle unit with a theoretical $\dot{Q}m/\dot{V}O_2m$ <6 will have increased anaerobic metabolism and lactate production. See text and Table 1 for application of model. Modified from Wasserman.[17]

tional unit. The muscle nourished by blood in which the $ccPO_2$ had been reached must obtain its ATP from anaerobic glycolysis (Fig. 5, pathway B). Since the $ccPO_2$ is the lowest capillary PO_2 in the capillary bed, the lowest muscle venous PO_2 during exercise would closely approximate the $ccPO_2$.

The fall in capillary PO_2 along the muscle-capillary bed can be predicted from the muscle blood flow/metabolic rate ratio ($\dot{Q}m/\dot{V}O_2m$), the arterial PO_2, the concentration of hemoglobin, the shape of the oxyhemoglobin dissociation curve, and the Bohr effect. The model shown in Figure 7 assumes a hemoglobin concentration of 15 g/dL, that arterial PO_2 is 90 mm Hg, that the rate of O_2 consumption along the capillary bed is constant, and that the Bohr effect is limited to the CO_2 produced as a result of aerobic metabolism.[17] Given these values, each liter of blood will contain 200 mL of O_2. If it were possible to completely extract O_2 from the blood, i.e., the $ccPO_2$ could fall to zero, the muscle could contract totally aerobically with a $\dot{Q}m/\dot{V}O_2m = 5$. But, of course, this is impossible because a partial pressure gradient must exist to allow O_2 to flow from the capillary (O_2 source) to the mitochondria (O_2 sink). Experimentally, the maximal extraction of O_2 from muscle-capillary blood during peak exercise is about 85%, as estimated from femoral venous and arterial blood.[18] To achieve this, the blood flow to the legs must be at least 6 L/min to perform a work task with a muscle $\dot{V}O_2 = 1$ L/min, i.e., consumption of five sixths of the O_2 transported to muscle.[19,20] The blood flow requirement must be even higher in patients with arterial hypoxemia, anemia, or carboxyhemoglobinemia.

If skeletal muscle O_2 consumption increases faster than its blood flow, the end-capillary PO_2, as approximated by the femoral venous PO_2, must decrease. When the capillary PO_2 cannot overcome the diffusive resistance between the capillary red cell and mitochondria to sustain aerobic regeneration of ATP, the capillary PO_2 would have fallen to its lowest ("critical") value. This would be first detected at the venous end of the capillary or in the venous effluent blood of the muscle, as a failure for end-capillary PO_2 to decrease further despite increasing $\dot{V}O_2$ (Fig. 8).[18,21]

Capillary PO₂, Critical Capillary PO₂, and Mean Capillary PO₂

The capillary PO_2 falls as blood traverses the capillary from arterial to venous end. The effect of the $\dot{Q}m/\dot{V}O_2m$ ratio on the decrease in PO_2 along the capillary bed has been described.[17,22] Muscle metabolic units at the arterial end of the capillary bed enjoy a high PO_2 partial pressure gradient and therefore do not require anaerobic glycolysis to regenerate ATP; but muscle metabolic units exposed to capillary blood toward the venous end may experience critical levels of hypoxia and undergo anaerobic metabolism. The rate of fall in capillary PO_2 as blood flows through the capillary bed and the point in the capillary bed at which the capillary PO_2 reaches the $ccPO_2$ are determined by the $\dot{Q}m/\dot{V}O_2m$ ratio. PO_2 will stop decreasing along the capillary bed if the $ccPO_2$ is reached before the end of the capillary. As illustrated by the curves for $\dot{Q}m/\dot{V}O_2m = 5$, 4, and 3 in Figure 7, the lower the $\dot{Q}m/\dot{V}O_2m$, the further toward the arterial end of the capillary that the $ccPO_2$ would be reached. Assuming a uniform $\dot{Q}m/\dot{V}O_2m$ ratio of 6, a normal hemoglobin concentration, and a $ccPO_2 = 16$, anaerobic glycolysis with net lactic acid production will likely not take place or would be slight. In contrast, as $\dot{Q}m/\dot{V}O_2m$ falls below 6, O_2 flow from red cell to myocyte must either decrease below 16, or if 16 is the $ccPO_2$, it must function partially anaerobically. In the latter case, lactate will increase in the venous effluent blood.

Aerobic metabolism of glycogen regenerates 3 mmol of ATP at the cost of a half mmol or 11.2 mL of O_2. Regenerating the same number of ATP

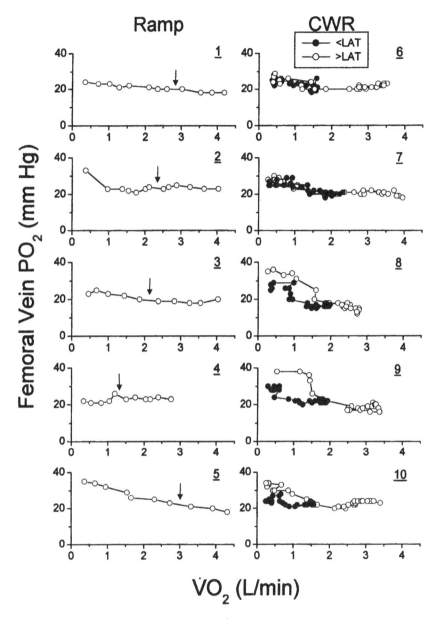

Figure 8. Femoral vein PO_2 as a function of $\dot{V}O_2$ for 5 normal subjects during a progressively increasing work rate test (left column) and 5 different normal subjects during two constant work rate tests, one moderate (solid circles) and one heavy (open circles). The down arrows in the left column indicate the anaerobic threshold $\dot{V}O_2$ in the respective study. CWR = constant work rate. Modified from Stringer et al.[18]

from anaerobic metabolism of glycogen produces 2 mmol of lactate and 2 mmol of CO_2 as 2 mmol of HCO_3^- buffer the 2 mmol of lactic acid. On a mmol-for-mmol basis, to produce the same number of ATP by anaerobic metabolism as by aerobic metabolism, with a glycosyl component of glycogen as the substrate, 4 mmol of lactate and CO_2 are produced for every 1 mmol reduction in O_2 consumed (6 mmol of lactate to 1 mmol of O_2 if glucose were the substrate).

The effect of the $\dot{Q}m/\dot{V}O_2m$ ratio distribution in four muscle models on muscle $\dot{V}O_2$, venous (femoral vein) PO_2, total muscle blood flow, and lactate production for a work rate requiring a steady state $\dot{V}O_2$ of 1.5 L/min is shown in Table 1. Each model is limited to three functional muscle units, each requiring one third of the total ATP regeneration. If the three muscle units had a uniformly high $\dot{Q}m/\dot{V}O_2m$, e.g., 8 (Model 1), it would be overperfused (12 L/min) and have a femoral venous PO_2 above the $ccPO_2$ (25), and $\dot{V}O_2 = 1.5$ L/min. Thus, there would be no net lactate production. Similarly, if the muscle units had a uniform $\dot{Q}m/\dot{V}O_2m = 6$ (Model 2), there would be no net increase in lactate production because the capillary PO_2 would not decrease to the $ccPO_2$ until the blood reached the end of the capillary of the metabolic unit. Muscle blood flow of Model 2 would be 9.0 L/min and $\dot{V}O_2 = 1.5$ L/min. However, if the muscle units had a uniform $\dot{Q}m/\dot{V}O_2m = 5$ (Model 3), i.e., $1\frac{1}{2}$ L/min less blood flow than required for the muscle to function totally aerobically, the $ccPO_2$ would be reached at a point 80% of the distance between the artery and the vein. Because the last fifth of the muscle would have to function anaerobically, it would be necessary to increase lactate production by 18 mmol/min from each of the three muscle components to compensate anaerobically for the aerobic deficit (0.1 L/min O_2 for each muscle component) (Table 1). In contrast, if the three muscle units had a nonuniform $\dot{Q}m/\dot{V}O_2m$ ratio distribution, e.g., combination of $\dot{Q}m/\dot{V}O_2m = 8$, 6, and 5 (Model 4), there would be a total O_2 deficit of 0.1 L/min for the exercise. This difference in O_2 deficit would be very difficult to detect (a $\dot{V}O_2 = 1.4$ L/min instead of 1.5 L/min), but the increase in lactate would be very easily measured, as hypothesized by the model of Whipp et al.[23] The uneven $\dot{Q}m/\dot{V}O_2m$ of Model 4 would result in increased lactate efflux from the muscle despite an increase in total blood flow greater than for Model 2 (9.5 vs. 9.0 L/min). End-capillary (femoral vein) PO_2 will increase to 20 instead of the 16 shown for Models 2 and 3. Koike et al.[21] found this paradoxical increase in femoral venous PO_2, with increase in lactate as $\dot{V}O_2$ increased, to be not uncommon in heart failure patients.

The observation that the normal cardiac output increase in response to exercise (i.e., $\Delta Q/\Delta\dot{V}O_2$) is approximately 6 L/min per liter of $\dot{V}O_2$[19,20] suggests that good matching of perfusion to metabolism is a normal phenomenon. The model presented in Figure 7 shows that if $\dot{Q}m/\dot{V}O_2m$ shifts to a lower ratio line than 6, the "mean" capillary PO_2 would decrease without a change in muscle venous effluent PO_2. Thus, a mean partial pressure

Table 1

Lactate Efflux from Muscle for Four Models of $\dot{Q}m/\dot{V}o_2m$ Ratios for Exercise Requiring a Steady State $\dot{V}o_2 = 1.5$ L/min

State of $\dot{Q}m/\dot{V}o_2m$	$\dot{Q}m/\dot{V}o_2m$			$\dot{V}o_2$ (L/min)			Fem. Vein PO_2 (mm Hg)	Tot. Blood Flow (L/min)	Lactate Efflux (mmol/min)		
	A	B	C	A	B	C			A	B	C
Model 1	8	8	8	0.5	0.5	0.5	25	12.0	0.0	0.0	0.0
Model 2	6	6	6	0.5	0.5	0.5	16	9.0	0.0	0.0	0.0
Model 3	5	5	5	0.4	0.4	0.4	16	7.5	18.0	18.0	18.0
Model 4	8	6	5	0.5	0.5	0.4	20	9.5	0.0	0.0	18.0

A, B, and C are three muscle components, each doing one third of the work.

gradient between the capillary and myocyte, calculated from femoral vein PO_2 measurements, would not be correct for work rates above the *AT*.

Measurement of Critical Capillary PO_2

Stringer et al.[18] and Koike et al.[21] showed that femoral vein PO_2, a surrogate of muscle end-capillary PO_2, does not continually decrease as $\dot{V}O_2$ increases. Figure 8 shows the femoral vein PO_2 measurements for the subjects in the report by Stringer et al.[18] in which measurements were made during increasing work rate (Ramp) in 5 normal subjects and constant work rate (CWR) exercise tests below and above the *AT* in 5 additional normal subjects. The right panels of Figure 8, illustrating the results of the two CWR tests, show reproducibility of femoral vein PO_2 measurements for different work rate protocols for a given subject. This reproducibility in femoral vein PO_2 was also shown by the investigation of Koike et al.[21] in which three exercise studies were done on each of 10 patients with chronic heart failure (CHF). That investigation also showed that the trough (critical capillary) PO_2 for each subject was consistent and achieved by the time the subjects developed a lactic acidosis.

The femoral vein lactate concentration was plotted as a function of femoral vein PO_2 in 10 healthy adults during upright cycle ergometer '"Ramp" and CWR exercise for normal subjects to determine the $ccPO_2$ (Fig. 9). During both the "Ramp" and the CWR exercise, femoral vein blood PO_2 reached a "floor" or lowest value ($ccPO_2$) before the lactate concentration started to increase (Fig. 9).[18] The femoral venous lactate concentration increased after the femoral venous and therefore the end-capillary PO_2 reached its lowest ($ccPO_2$) value. This ranged between 15 and 23 mm Hg. Similar findings were reported by Koike et al.[21] in patients with CHF. This observation in normal subjects and heart failure patients is predicted from the $ccPO_2$ theory and provides the dynamic link between minimal capillary PO_2, blood lactate increase, and the *AT* concept.

The O_2 Flow-Independent and O_2 Flow-Dependent Work Rate Zones and the *AT*

The *AT* concept implies that there is an exercise $\dot{V}O_2$ below which exercise $\dot{V}O_2$ is determined by the work rate performed and not the O_2 transport to the muscles and above which $\dot{V}O_2$ is determined by O_2 transport as well as the work rate. In other words, $\dot{V}O_2$ is O_2 flow independent below the *AT*, and $\dot{V}O_2$ is O_2 flow dependent above the *AT*. To test this hypothesis, Hansen et al.[24] increased work rate at slow, medium, and fast rates and found that $\dot{V}O_2$ increased at a rate that did not vary as the rate of increase in work rate

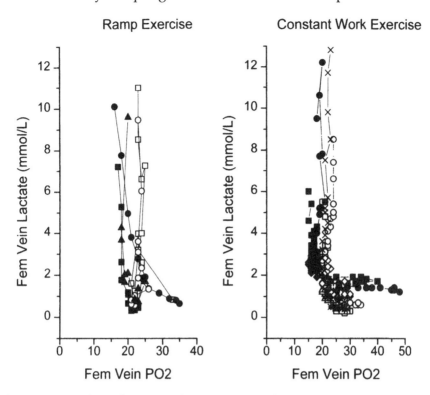

Figure 9. Femoral vein lactate as a function of femoral vein PO_2 for 5 normal subjects during a progressively increasing work rate test (Ramp) and 5 normal subjects during two constant work rate cycle ergometer exercise tests. The start of exercise is the most right point for the respective study. As exercise progresses, the PO_2 moves leftward to its minimal (critical) value at which level lactate starts to increase. From Stringer et al.[18]

varied below the *AT* in contrast to the rate of work rate increase above the *AT* (Fig. 10); however, peak $\dot{V}O_2$ was unchanged.

The failure of $\dot{V}O_2$ to fully track work rate change above the *AT* was also shown by Haouzi et al.,[25] who changed work rate in sine wave pattern below and above the *AT* (Fig. 11). Below the *AT*, the amplitude in $\dot{V}O_2$ for a work rate period of 4 minutes varied with the amplitude of work rate in an approximate ratio of 10 mL/min/W. In contrast, the amplitude of change in $\dot{V}O_2$ for the same period and work rate change above the *AT* is only about two thirds as much, showing that above the *AT* the $\dot{V}O_2$ cannot fully respond to the O_2 requirement, i.e., is in the O_2 flow-dependent zone of work rate.

In studies in which blood O_2 content was decreased in a controlled fashion in normal subjects (Fig. 12), Koike et al.[10,26] also demonstrated that the *AT* demarcates the O_2 flow-independent from the O_2 flow-dependent work rate zones. In these studies, blood O_2 content was reduced by taking up O_2 binding sites on hemoglobin with carbon monoxide to reduce blood O_2 content by approximately 10% and 20% before performing exercise. The *AT* and peak $\dot{V}O_2$ were reduced by a percentage, consistent with the percent

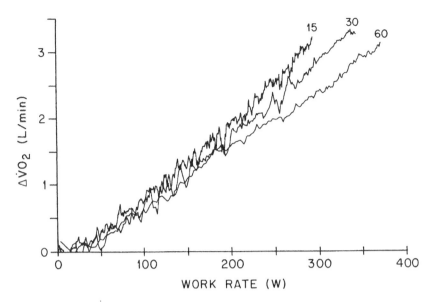

Figure 10. Effect of rate of increase in work rate from unloaded cycling on rate of increase in $\dot{V}O_2$ in a normal subject. Below the anaerobic threshold work rate (approx. 180 W), the rate of increase in $\dot{V}O_2$ is independent of the rate of increase in work rate. The faster the rate of increase in work rate, the slower the increase in $\dot{V}O_2$ above the anaerobic threshold, although the peak $\dot{V}O_2$ is unchanged. From Hansen et al.[24]

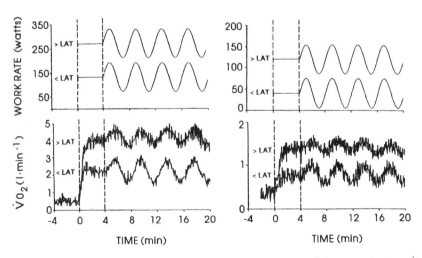

Figure 11. Effect of continuously changing work rate in sinusoidal pattern (top) on $\dot{V}O_2$ kinetics (bottom) for a range of changing work rate below (< LAT) and above (> LAT) the lactic acidosis (anaerobic) threshold for two normal subjects. From Haouzi et al.[25]

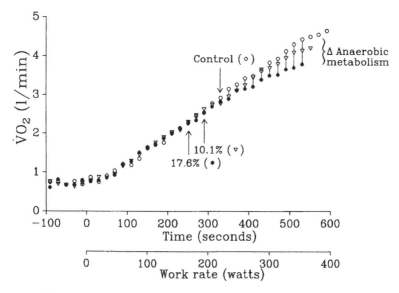

Figure 12. Effect of reducing blood O_2 content by increasing blood carboxyhemoglobin (COHb) concentration on $\dot{V}O_2$, anaerobic threshold (AT, arrows), and peak $\dot{V}O_2$ in a normal subject repeating the same work rate protocol. Each study was done on a separate day. In one study the subject breathed pure air (control) and was not preloaded with COHb. In a second study the subject breathed 0.2% CO before exercise to increase the subject's COHb to 10.1% and then breathed 0.02% CO during exercise to maintain the COHb concentration. The same exercise test was repeated a third time on a different day except that the subject breathed the 0.2% CO longer before the exercise test to increase the COHb concentration to 17.6% and then maintained at that level by 0.02% CO breathing during exercise. The order of tests was random. There was no effect on $\dot{V}O_2$ as work rate was increased until the AT (arrow) of the respective study was surpassed. Then the increase in $\dot{V}O_2$ was slower the higher the COHb. The difference between the $\dot{V}O_2$ of the control and the reduced blood O_2 content studies represents the reduced $\dot{V}O_2$ caused by the reduced blood O_2 content. The AT and peak $\dot{V}O_2$ were systematically reduced as the blood O_2 content was decreased.

reduction in blood O_2 content. While $\dot{V}O_2$ increased at an unchanged rate for different levels of carboxyhemoglobin at the work rates below the AT, the rate of increase in $\dot{V}O_2$ was reduced for the work rates above the AT.

Pattern of Capillary Recruitment:
Diffusion-Limited and Non-Diffusion-Limited
O_2 Consumption

In a recent review, Wagner[27] discussed the effect of the diffusional conductance of O_2 in muscle on $\dot{V}O_2$max. Diffusion-limited O_2 consumption is present when capillary PO_2 can decrease no further despite increasing $\dot{V}O_2$. The venous end of the capillary must be the earliest site of diffusion-

$$\dot{V}O_2 = DxA/LxP(c-m)O_2$$

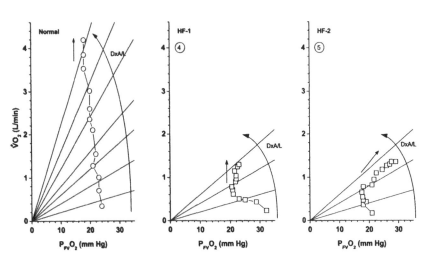

Figure 13. Pattern of change in $\dot{V}O_2$ as a function of femoral vein (end-capillary) PO_2 in a normal subject (left) and in two heart failure patients (center and right). The slopes radiating from the origin are the product of the diffusion coefficient for O_2 (D) and the capillary surface area (A) divided by the diffusion distance (L) (see Fick law of diffusion equation on top). As $\dot{V}O_2$ increases, PO_2 eventually reaches a minimal (critical) value. This would reflect the minimal end-capillary-mitochondrial PO_2 difference [P(c-m)O_2] assuming mitochondrial PO_2 functions at about 1 mm Hg. The normal subjects and patients have a similar minimal femoral vein PO_2 but at different $\dot{V}O_2$ values. The femoral vein PO_2, reflecting the end-capillary PO_2, changes in two different ways in heart failure patients. It either remains essentially constant, as in normal subjects (HF I), or increases (HF II). In HF II, end-capillary PO_2 increases with increasing $\dot{V}O_2$ after reaching its nadir. When femoral vein PO_2 reaches its critical (minimal) value, increasing $\dot{V}O_2$ must be diffusion limited (follows the Fick law for a diffusion-limited process). The arrows indicate the direction of increasing work rate. Data taken from Stringer et al.[18] and Koike et al.[21]

limited muscle O_2 consumption. In contrast, the O_2 consumption in the region of the myocyte near the arterial end of the capillary should virtually never be diffusion limited. From the Fick law of diffusion (Fig. 13), the only mechanism to account for the increase in $\dot{V}O_2$, while end-capillary PO_2 remains constant, is for the diffusion surface area (A) to increase and/or diffusion distance (L) to decrease (diffusion-limited capillary recruitment). In addition, the exercise lactic acidosis that develops once the ccPO_2 is reached facilitates further dissociation of O_2 from hemoglobin (Bohr effect),[18] allowing muscle $\dot{V}O_2$ to increase without a further decrease in capillary PO_2.

The pattern of increase in $\dot{V}O_2$ as related to end-capillary or femoral vein PO_2 provides insight into the range of work that is non-diffusion-limited $\dot{V}O_2$ and the range of work rate that is diffusion-limited $\dot{V}O_2$ (Fig. 13). From the Fick law of diffusion, diffusion-limited $\dot{V}O_2$ is directly proportional to the capillary-mitochondrial PO_2 gradient. In contrast, an inverse relationship between increasing $\dot{V}O_2$ and capillary-mitochondrial PO_2 gradient defies the Fick law of diffusion, and therefore increasing $\dot{V}O_2$ must not be diffusion limited. Not until the capillary-mitochondrial PO_2 gradient stops decreasing, or increases, is $\dot{V}O_2$ likely to be diffusion limited.

If the mitochondrial PO_2 is assumed to be only about 1 mm Hg,[16] the end-capillary or femoral vein PO_2 must closely describe the $P(c-m)O_2$ at the region of the capillary where the PO_2 is most likely to be critical (venous end of the capillary). Figure 13 shows plots of increasing $\dot{V}O_2$ versus femoral vein PO_2 as work rate is increased for a fit normal subject (left) from the studies of Stringer et al.,[18] and two heart failure subjects (middle and right) from the study of Koike et al.[21] From the Fick diffusion equation, the slopes radiating from the origin must be the product of the diffusivity constant (D) and the O_2 diffusion surface area (A) divided by the diffusion distance (L), with A/L being a function of the muscle-capillary density. $\dot{V}O_2$ increasing while femoral vein PO_2 ($P_{FV}PO_2$) is decreasing (Fig. 13), is accounted for by non-diffusion-limited $\dot{V}O_2$. In contrast, when $P_{FV}PO_2$ is constant (left and middle) or increasing (right), $\dot{V}O_2$ must be diffusion limited. Thus, when femoral venous PO_2 stops decreasing as $\dot{V}O_2$ continues to increase, O_2 transfer to the myocyte changes from non-diffusion-limited to diffusion-limited $\dot{V}O_2$. The further increase in $\dot{V}O_2$ is attributable to an increase in A/L and/or the release of O_2 from hemoglobin because of blood acidification (Bohr effect).[18]

From the study of Koike et al.,[21] two different patterns of change in the $\dot{V}O_2$ versus $P_{FV}O_2$ were found in patients with CHF. These are replotted from the original published data in the center and right panels of Figure 13. The two patterns of $\dot{V}O_2$ increase as a function of $P_{FV}O_2$ are defined as HF I (Fig. 13, center panel) and HF II (Fig. 13, right panel). The heart failure patients had relatively little non-diffusion-limited capillary recruitment. In HF I patients, $P_{FV}O_2$ remained constant after reaching its $ccPO_2$. In contrast, $P_{FV}O_2$ increased at a $\dot{V}O_2$ above that at which the $ccPO_2$ was reached in the HF II patients, consistent with diffusion-limited muscle $\dot{V}O_2$.

Role of Exercise-Induced
Lactic Acidosis on $\dot{V}O_2$ and $\dot{V}CO_2$ Kinetics

The role of the lactic acidosis of above AT exercise affects the $\dot{V}O_2$ and $\dot{V}CO_2$ kinetics as shown in Figure 14. As soon as lactic acid production increases, it must be immediately buffered on its formation because lactic acid is virtually totally dissociated at the pH of the cell. The primary buffer for the lactic acid is HCO_3^-. Because 22.3 mL of CO_2 is produced from HCO_3^- buffering of 1 mmol of lactic acid, $\dot{V}CO_2$ increases substantially above that derived from aerobic regeneration of ATP.[17] This increase in $\dot{V}CO_2$ over that produced from aerobic metabolism accounts for a greater $\dot{V}CO_2$ than that for a subject performing the same work rate below the AT. The increase in

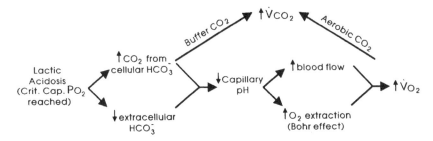

Figure 14. Hypothesis by which the rate of lactic acid accumulation during exercise affects O_2 uptake and CO_2 output. Above the lactic acidosis threshold, $\dot{V}_{CO_2}$ increases disproportionately to $\dot{V}_{O_2}$ depending on the rate of lactic acid accumulating in the body (upper chain of arrows). Simultaneously, there is an equimolar decrease in HCO_3^- to the increase in lactate and an increase in PCO_2 in the muscle (Fig. 6). Both decrease in HCO_3^- and increase in CO_2 production reduce the regional capillary pH. This decrease in pH increases regional blood flow and promotes oxyhemoglobin dissociation (Bohr effect) thereby allowing $\dot{V}_{O_2}$ to increase in proportion to the lactate increase. Reproduced from Wasserman.[17]

H^+ accompanying the exercise-induced lactic acidosis allows $\dot{V}_{O_2}$ to continue to increase by two mechanisms, capillary recruitment and the Bohr effect (Fig. 14). The regional lactic acidosis, or an associated metabolite, acts to vasodilate and recruit capillary surface area. Thus, capillary recruitment and O_2 transport are increased where anaerobiosis is greatest. This increase in O_2 availability allows $\dot{V}_{O_2}$ to increase in proportion to the increase in lactate.[17]

In addition to vasodilatation, the regional lactic acidosis shifts the oxyhemoglobin dissociation curve downward and to the right, facilitating the dissociation of O_2 from hemoglobin without a decrease in capillary PO_2.[18] This allows $\dot{V}_{O_2}$ to increase in proportion to the lactate increase in the O_2 flow-dependent work rate zone (above the AT).[28] From the dependency of muscle extraction of O_2 on the lactic acidosis of heavy exercise, the lactic acidosis can be viewed as an adaptation to facilitate cellular respiration and oxidative metabolism under conditions of relatively high O_2 requirement. Evidence that the lactic acidosis of exercise contributes to the muscle O_2 supply is revealed by studies on patients with muscle enzyme disorders that prevent lactate from increasing normally in response to exercise, such as in McArdle's syndrome.[29] These studies show that these patients[30] have an abnormally reduced peak $\dot{V}_{O_2}$ and greatly reduced arterial-venous O_2 difference at their maximally tolerated $\dot{V}_{O_2}$, suggesting that they cannot extract O_2 normally from the muscle blood flow.

Summary

The ability of the circulation to transport O_2 at the rate required by the muscles during exercise is a measure of cardiovascular health. The role of the circulation during exercise is to couple external to muscle respiration in order to aerobically regenerate ATP needed for muscle contraction.

Failure of the circulation to deliver O_2 at the rate needed during the first several minutes of exercise for aerobic regeneration of ATP results in anaerobic regeneration of ATP from hydrolysis of PCr. The PCr hydrolysis results in a transient metabolic alkalosis at the muscle site because creatine is a neutral molecule compared to the relatively highly dissociated PCr (acts as an acid) at cellular pH. Increases in pH and HCO_3^- in the femoral vein blood early during leg cycling exercise reveal this metabolic alkalosis. As a result of this reaction, $\dot{V}CO_2$ is reduced relative to $\dot{V}O_2$ during the early phase of exercise.

Failure to deliver adequate O_2 to the tissues also results in an inadequate rate of aerobic regeneration of ATP, reflected in slow $\dot{V}O_2$ kinetics and increased anaerobic glycolysis. Accompanying the latter is a second source of ATP regeneration, but it is generated at a high glycogen substrate cost. The byproduct of this reaction is a lactic acidosis. Because the lactic acid is buffered predominantly by HCO_3^-, $\dot{V}CO_2$ increases relative to $\dot{V}O_2$. This continues as long as lactate accumulates (production > removal). Thus, the patterns of $\dot{V}O_2$ and $\dot{V}CO_2$ differ during exercise depending on the magnitude of PCr hydrolysis and anaerobic glycolysis. The former reduces $\dot{V}CO_2$ primarily during the first minute or so of exercise and the latter increases $\dot{V}CO_2$ primarily after 1 minute of exercise.

Femoral vein PO_2 reaches its lowest value ($ccPO_2$) at approximately the mid level of the subject's work capacity, on average, not at $\dot{V}O_2max$. Muscle $\dot{V}O_2$ is not diffusion limited until femoral vein (end-capillary) PO_2 reaches its lowest value. Femoral vein lactate increases during leg cycling exercise after the $ccPO_2$ is reached. The increase in lactate is essential to continue exercise beyond the *anaerobic (lactic acidosis) threshold, AT,* because the H^+ that accompanies the lactate increase facilitates oxyhemoglobin dissociation. This is, functionally, a respiratory adaptation for anaerobiosis and may represent the most important role that lactic acidosis plays during heavy exercise.

Both normal subjects and patients with chronic stable heart failure have a similar $ccPO_2$ suggesting no significant defect in extraction of O_2 from blood in heart failure patients. The pattern of change in femoral vein (end-capillary) PO_2 as $\dot{V}O_2$ increases describes the $\dot{V}O_2$ at which O_2 becomes diffusion limited and the extent to which new muscle-capillary diffusion surface is recruited during exercise. While the $ccPO_2$ is similar in heart failure patients and normal subjects, the $\dot{V}O_2$ at which the $ccPO_2$ is reached is greatly reduced in heart failure. Thus, the $\dot{V}O_2$ at which the $ccPO_2$ is reached determines the onset of anaerobic glycolysis with increased lactate production. Consequently, the measurement of *AT* by gas exchange reveals the $\dot{V}O_2$ below which O_2 transport and consumption is sustainable without a lactic acidosis (steady state) and above which it is not. Thus, the *AT* is a valuable submaximal parameter of aerobic function, particularly when attempting to evaluate cardiovascular health.

References

1. McGilvery RW. Oxidations and phosphorylations. In: McGilvery RW (ed): Biochemistry: A Functional Approach. Philadelphia: W.B. Saunders Co.; 1983:390-420.
2. Bessman SP, Geiger PJ. Transport of energy in muscle: the phosphorylcreatine shuttle. Science 1981;211:448-452.
3. Barstow TJ, Buchthal S, Zanconato S, Cooper DM. Muscle energetics and pulmonary oxygen uptake kinetics during moderate exercise. J Appl Physiol 1994;74:1742-1749.
4. Rossiter HB, Ward SA, Doyle VL, Howe FA, Griffiths JR, Whipp BJ. Inferences from pulmonary O_2 uptake with respect to intramuscular [phosphocreatine] kinetics during moderate exercise in humans. J Physiol 1999;518(Pt. 3):921-932.
5. Yoshida T, Watari H. Changes in intracellular pH during repeated exercise. Eur J Appl Physiol 1993;67:274-278.
6. Adams GR, Foley JM, Meyer RA. Muscle buffer capacity estimated from pH changes during rest-to-work transitions. J Appl Physiol 1990;69:968-972.
7. Wasserman K, Stringer W, Casaburi R, Zhang YY. Mechanism of the exercise hyperkalemia: an alternate hypothesis. J Appl Physiol 1997;83:631-643.
8. Chuang M-L, Ting H, Otsuka T, Sun X-G, et al. Aerobically generated CO_2 stored during early exercise. J Appl Physiol 1999;87:1048-1058.
9. Connett RJ, Sahlin K. Control of glycolysis and glycogen metabolism. In: Rowell LB, Shepherd JT (eds): Exercise: Regulation and Integration of Multiple Systems. New York: Oxford University Press; Handbook of Physiology: Section 12. 1996:870-911.
10. Koike A, Weiler-Ravell D, McKenzie DK, Zanconato S, Wasserman K. Evidence that the metabolic acidosis threshold is the anaerobic threshold. J Appl Physiol 1990;68:2521-2526.
11. Koike A, Wasserman K, Taniguichi K, Hiroe M, Marumo F. The critical capillary PO_2 and the lactate threshold in patients with cardiovascular disease. J Am Coll Cardiol 1994;23:1644-1650.
12. Wasserman K, Whipp BJ, Koyal S, Beaver WL. Anaerobic threshold and respiratory gas exchange during exercise. J Appl Physiol 1973;35:236-243.
13. Beaver WL, Wasserman K, Whipp BJ. A new method for detecting the anaerobic threshold by gas exchange. J Appl Physiol 1986;60:2020-2027.
14. Wasserman K, Beaver WL, Davis JA, Pu J-Z, Heber D, Whipp BJ. Lactate, pyruvate, and lactate-to-pyruvate ratio during exercise and recovery. J Appl Physiol 1985;59:935-940.
15. Wittenberg BA, Wittenberg JB. Transport of oxygen in muscle. Ann Rev Physiol 1989;51:857-878.
16. Chance B, Williams GR. Respiratory enzymes in oxidative phosphorylation. J Biol Chem 1955;217:383-393.
17. Wasserman K. Coupling of external to cellular respiration during exercise: the wisdom of the body revisited. Am J Physiol 1994;266:E519-E539.
18. Stringer W, Wasserman K, Casaburi R, Porszasz J, Maehara K, French W. Lactic acidosis as a facilitator of oxyhemoglobin dissociation during exercise. J Appl Physiol 1994;76:1462-1467.
19. Rowell LB. Human Circulation Regulation During Physical Stress. New York: Oxford University Press; 1986:215.

20. Weber KT, Janicki JS. Cardiopulmonary Exercise Testing: Physiological Principles and Clinical Applications. Philadelphia: W.B. Saunders Co.; 1986:238-243.

21. Koike A, Wasserman K, Taniguichi K, Hiroe M, Marumo F. Critical capillary oxygen partial pressure and lactate threshold in patients with cardiovascular disease. J Am Coll Cardiol 1994;23:1644-1650.

22. Wasserman K, Stringer W. Critical capillary PO_2, net lactate production, and oxyhemoglobin dissociation: effects on exercise gas exchange. In: Wasserman K (ed): Exercise Gas Exchange in Heart Disease. Armonk, NY: Futura Publishing Co.; 1996:157-181.

23. Whipp BJ, Lamarra N, Ward SA. Obligatory anaerobiosis resulting from oxygen uptake-to-blood flow ratio dispersion in skeletal muscle: a model. Eur J Appl Physiol Occup Physiol 1995;71:147-152.

24. Hansen JE, Sue DY, Oren A, Wasserman K. Relation of oxygen uptake in work rate in normal men and men with circulatory disorders. Am J Cardiol 1987;59:669-674.

25. Haouzi P, Fukuba Y, Casaburi R, Stringer W, Wasserman K. O_2 uptake kinetics above and below the lactic acidosis threshold during sinusoidal exercise. J Appl Physiol 1993;75:1644-1650.

26. Koike A, Wasserman K, McKenzie DK, Zanconato S, Weiler-Ravell D. Evidence that diffusion limitation determines oxygen uptake kinetics during exercise in humans. J Clin Invest 1990;86:1698-1706.

27. Wagner PD. Diffusive resistance to O_2 transport in muscle. Acta Physiol Scand 2000;168:609-614.

28. Wasserman K, Hansen J, Sue DY, Casaburi R, Whipp BJ. Principles of Exercise Testing and Interpretation. 3rd ed. Baltimore: Lippincott, Williams and Wilkins; 1999:19-43.

29. Lewis SF, Haller RG. The pathophysiology of McArdle's disease: clues to regulation in exercise and fatigue. J Appl Physiol 1986;61:391-401.

30. Lewis SF, Vora S, Haller RG. Abnormal oxidative metabolism and O_2 transport in muscle phosphofructokinase deficiency. J Appl Physiol 1991;70:391-398.

2

Skeletal Muscle Metabolism During Exercise in Chronic Heart Failure

Koichi Okita, MD

Exercise tolerance is impaired in patients with chronic heart failure (CHF). Traditionally, exercise intolerance was thought to be related to central hemodynamic disturbance in patients with CHF; however, recent studies have reported that skeletal muscle abnormalities are important contributors to exercise intolerance.[1-14] This chapter presents the three studies done by our group that concern skeletal muscle metabolism in patients with CHF.

Skeletal Muscle Metabolism During Localized Exercise in Patients with CHF

In the last decade, several studies showed that skeletal muscle abnormalities such as reductions in skeletal muscle mass, aerobic enzyme activity, and mitochondrial volume, and an increased percentage of fast-twitch (IIb) fibers were seen in the skeletal muscle of patients with CHF. These abnormalities can induce early anaerobic metabolism during exercise and may limit exercise capacity.[1,5-9,11] These findings have been confirmed in localized muscle exercise of the forearm or calf by studies using ^{31}P magnetic resonance spectroscopy (^{31}P-MRS).[2-4,7,10] We discuss here the study of muscle metabolism during localized muscle exercise. In this study, we measured muscle metabolism of both the forearm and the calf in each patient and control.

From Wasserman K (ed): *Cardiopulmonary Exercise Testing and Cardiovascular Health.* Armonk, NY: Futura Publishing Company, Inc.; © 2002.

Methods

We studied 13 patients with CHF and 11 age- and size-matched normal subjects (Table 1). Before participation in the study, subjects underwent examinations to detect peripheral vascular diseases including palpation of peripheral pulses. Informed consent was obtained from all subjects.

^{31}P-MRS was performed using an 80-mm surface coil in a 55-cm bore and a 1.5-T superconducting magnet (Magnetom H15, Siemens Medical Systems, Germany). Shimming was adjusted by using the proton signal from water. Spectra were obtained with a pulse width of 500 ms, a transmitter voltage of 20.0 V, and a repetition time of 2000 ms. Each spectrum represented the average of 16 scans. One measurement required about 40 seconds. Since only the relative changes in high-energy phosphates were evaluated, we did not correct values for saturation. Phosphocreatine (PCr) was standardized as follows: $[PCr]/([PCr]+[Pi])$, where Pi is inorganic phosphate. The muscle pH was calculated from changes in the chemical shifts of Pi relative to PCr ($pH = 6.75 + \log [(s-3.27)/(5.69-s)]$: $s(ppm) = Pi-PCr$).[14-17]

In order to load a subject, we set a pulley system to the whole-body magnetic resonance system. The supine unilateral plantar flexion or forearm flexion was performed with a multistage incremental protocol (Fig. 1). Protocols for the forearm and the calf were the same.[14,15] We normalized the workload to adjust for differences in muscle mass. First, we measured the maximal cross-sectional area (MCA) of the flexor muscles in each subject using magnetic resonance imaging (MRI). Recruited muscles in the exercise protocol were determined by T2-weighted MRI in another experiment.[18] The subject's right arm or calf was placed on a pedal attached via a pulley system to loads. The load was initially set at 0.05 kg/cm^2 of the MCA and was

___ **Table 1** ___

Baseline Characteristics of Normal Controls and Patients with Chronic Heart Failure (Study 1)

	Normal Controls	Patients with CHF
Subject (n)	11	13
Male (n)	6	7
Female (n)	5	6
Age (yr)	49±6	52±12
Height (cm)	158±7	161±8
Weight (kg)	54±6	59±8
NYHA functional class (n)		
II		7
III		6
Peak V̇O$_2$ (mL/kg/min)	30.9±6.5	18.9±4.4*
AT (mL/kg/min)	21.5±4.3	13.9±2.9*

CHF = chronic heart failure; NYHA = New York Heart Association. All values are the mean±SD.*p<0.0001 versus controls.

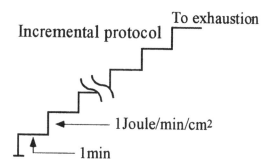

Figure 1. Protocol for localized muscle exercise.

increased by 0.05 kg/cm² every minute. The load was lifted 5 cm each time and the lifting was repeated 40 times/min. Thus, the workload is equal to 1 J/min/cm². During exercise, the subject's muscle metabolism was measured by ^{31}P-MRS every minute. To evaluate the metabolic capacity during calf plantar flexion and forearm wrist flexion, we calculated the slope of the PCr decrease in relation to increases in the workload by linear regression (PC-slope). Since PCr decreases linearly in response to a progressively increasing workload, the PC-slope is a simple indicator of the rate of PCr breakdown against the workload, which may mainly reflect the oxidative capacity of skeletal muscle. We used the muscle pH at the submaximal workload to evaluate muscle acidification. In this study submaximal was determined to be 70% of the maximal work rate. Systemic exercise capacity was derived with an upright bicycle ergometer (Corival 400, Lode, Holland) using a ramp protocol. Respiratory gas analysis was performed using a breath-by-breath apparatus (Aeromonitor AE-280, Minato Medical Science, Osaka, Japan). The gas exchange anaerobic threshold (*AT*) was determined by the V-slope method, as described by Wasserman et al.[19]

Results

There were no statistical differences in forearm and calf sizes between patients and controls (Table 2). There was, however, a significant difference in the proportion of forearm to calf size. This would mean that the calf muscle was relatively atrophied compared to the forearm in patients with CHF. In both muscles there was no statistically significant difference in the maximal work rate normalized by muscle mass between patients and controls.

Figure 2 shows the time course of changes in PCr and muscle pH during calf plantar flexion. The PCr and muscle pH decreased more rapidly as the workload increased in patients than in controls. Patients with CHF performed at a nearly normal maximal work rate accompanied by an enhanced anaerobic metabolism.

_____ **Table 2** _____

Results from Localized Muscle Exercise (Study 1)

	Normal Controls	Patients with CHF	Significance
Forearm MCA (cm^2)	13.0±3.8	15.8±3.1	ns
Calf MCA (cm^2)	41.5±8.6	38.6±4.8	ns
Ratio of forearm to calf	0.31±0.04	0.42±0.11	p<0.01
Maximal forearm work rate (J)	6.6±1.3	5.8±1.0	ns
Maximal calf work rate (J)	7.3±0.8	6.6±1.0	ns
PCr-slope of forearm	−0.060±0.025	−0.074±0.030	ns
PCr-slope of calf	−0.064±0.016	−0.082±0.019	p<0.05
Forearm muscle pH at the submaximal work rate	6.78±0.19	6.70±0.27	ns
Calf muscle pH at the submaximal work rate	7.04±0.05	6.89±0.06	p<0.0001

CHF = chronic heart failure; MCA = maximal cross-sectional area.

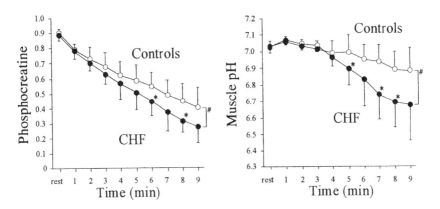

Figure 2. Time course of changes in phosphocreatine (PCr) and muscle pH during calf plantar flexion with the incremental protocol. The PCr and pH decreased more rapidly versus work rate in chronic heart failure (CHF) patients than in controls. *p<0.05 by Student's *t* test, #p<0.05 by analysis of variance versus controls.

The calculated PC-slope was steeper in patients than in controls in both muscles (Table 2), but a significant difference was seen only in the calf. There was a significant correlation between metabolic capacity evaluated as PC-slope and peak O_2 uptake (peak $\dot{V}O_2$) in each muscle (Fig. 3). There was also a significant correlation between PC-slope and gas exchange *AT* in the calf muscle (r=0.80, p<0.0001) but not in the forearm muscle (r=0.42, p=0.06).

There was a significant difference in muscle pH at the submaximal work rate (70% of maximal work rate) in the calf between patients and controls, but not in the forearm (Table 2). A lower muscle pH at the submaximal work rate indicates an earlier onset of anaerobic metabolism. There was a

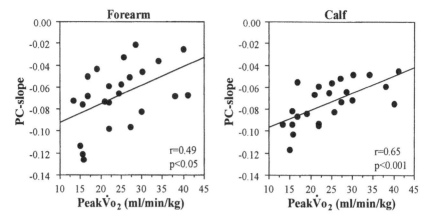

Figure 3. The relationship between metabolic capacity evaluated as PC-slope and peak O_2 uptake (peak $\dot{V}O_2$) in the forearm and calf.

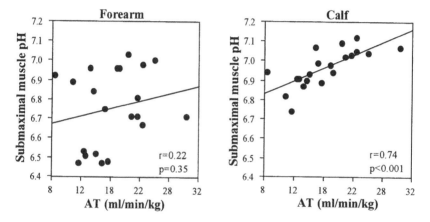

Figure 4. The relationship between muscle acidification evaluated as the muscle pH at the submaximal work rate and gas exchange anaerobic threshold (AT) in the forearm and calf.

significant correlation between muscle pH at the submaximal work rate and peak $\dot{V}O_2$ in the calf (r=0.78, p<0.0001), but not in the forearm (r=0.31, p= 0.14). There was also a significant correlation between muscle pH at the submaximal work rate and gas exchange *AT* in the calf muscle but not in the forearm (Fig. 4).

Conclusions

Impaired skeletal muscle metabolism during exercise is seen in the lower and the upper limbs in patients with CHF, with muscle metabolic abnormalities being more prominent in the lower limbs than in the upper limbs in these patients. Muscle abnormalities, especially in the lower limbs, are related to systemic exercise tolerance. Possible reasons for the different results between the forearm and calf are: 1) The difference in muscle mass between them. The larger the muscle mass, the more muscle metabolism is governed by muscle blood flow. 2) The difference in fiber type distribution between the forearm and calf. Forearm muscles might be composed of a large individual variety of fiber types, which might make the difference in muscle metabolism between controls and patients undetectable. 3) Muscle deconditioning might be greater in the lower limbs than in the upper limbs. 4) Systemic exercise capacity is measured during lower limb exercise. If the peak $\dot{V}O_2$ and AT were measured with an arm ergometer, a different picture might emerge.

Skeletal Muscle Metabolism During Systemic Exercise

Does skeletal muscle metabolism contribute to systemic exercise capacity? Results from ^{31}P-MRS studies were based on local exercises involving only a small muscle mass (the unilateral forearm or calf).[2-4,7,10] Whether the metabolic abnormalities observed with such a local exercise are also associated with systemic exercise and whether the muscle metabolism affects systemic exercise capacity have not been clarified. Thus, we attempted to measure skeletal muscle metabolism during systemic exercise and to investigate the effect of muscle metabolism on exercise tolerance. There are technical difficulties in performing ^{31}P-MRS during systemic exercise, such as an upright bicycle, mainly because of the small magnetic resonance bore size. Therefore, we chose the metabolic freeze method to stop the metabolism.[20,21] This method was first described by Harris et al.[20] in 1976. When the circulation to the working muscle is suddenly stopped by a cuff simultaneously with the cessation of exercise, the metabolism is "frozen" for at least several minutes and is preserved as it was during exercise. Only after the circulation is restored does metabolic recovery occur. We have confirmed the validity of the metabolic freeze method in a previous study.[12]

Methods

We studied 12 Japanese male patients with CHF and 7 age- and size-matched normal male subjects (Table 3). None of the patients had peripheral vascular disease. Informed consent was obtained from all subjects.

First, we placed a cuff around the thigh of each subject and performed a resting measurement. Next, the subject performed maximal upright bicycle exercise outside of the MRI apparatus. As soon as the subject indicated that he could not continue, he was asked to stop pedaling suddenly and the cuff

_____ Table 3 _____

Baseline Characteristics of Normal Controls and Patients with Chronic Heart Failure (Study 2)

	Normal Controls	Patients with CHF
Subject (n)	7	12
Age (yr)	50±7	57±8
Height (cm)	168±6	167±2
Weight (kg)	64±3	65±6
NYHA functional class		
II		7
III		5
Dilated cardiomyopathy		10
Ischemic heart disease		2
Atrial fibrillation		4
Peak $\dot{V}O_2$ (mL/kg/min)	31.8±3.7	20.2±3.0*
AT (mL/kg/min)	22.3±2.5	14.3±2.4*
LVEF (%)		0.23±0.10
Beta-blockers		4

AT = anaerobic threshold; CHF = chronic heart failure; LVEF = left ventricular ejection fraction; NYHA = New York Heart Association. All values are the mean±SD. *p<0.0001 versus controls. From Okita et al., Skeletal muscle metabolism limits exercise capacity in patients with chronic heart failure. Circulation 1998;98:1886-1891. Lippincott Williams & Wilkins.©

was simultaneously inflated to a suprasystolic pressure. The subject was then transferred to the MRI apparatus and ^{31}P-MRS was started immediately. The interval between the cessation of exercise and the start of measurement was usually 1 to 2 minutes.

To document the time course of the PCr and muscle pH changes in response to the increased workload with this method, the metabolic freeze was employed at various workloads during bicycle exercise in 2 patients and 2 controls. The PCr decreased linearly with increasing workloads (Fig. 5). Thus, we calculated the slope of the relation between the power output and the PCr decrease (Sys-slope) to evaluate metabolic capacity.

We also evaluated metabolic capacity during plantar flexion in each subject using the same method used in the former study. The capacity was described as the Loc-slope (the slope of the PCr decrease in relation to increases in the workload during plantar flexion).

Results

Figure 6 shows muscle metabolism during the peak exercise in both groups. The PCr was nearly depleted at this point in both groups. Muscle pH was more severely decreased in the patients than in the controls. These findings suggest that metabolic limitation coincides with the end of exercise. Metabolic limitation occurred at a significantly lower peak workload and $\dot{V}O_2$ in patients than in controls. Muscle metabolic capacity evaluated as the

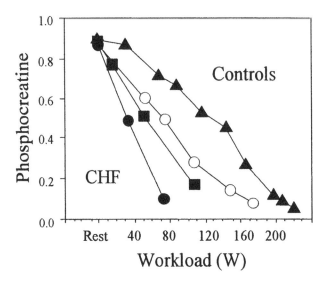

Figure 5. Time course of phosphocreatine change in response to increased workload during upright bicycle exercise in 2 patients with chronic heart failure (CHF; solid circles and squares) and controls (open circles and solid triangles).

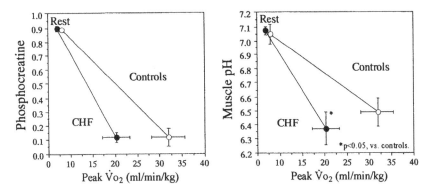

Figure 6. Phosphocreatine and muscle pH decrease during maximal bicycle exercise in patients with chronic heart failure (CHF) and controls.

Sys-slope was significantly correlated with the peak $\dot{V}_{O_2}$ and the AT (Fig. 7).

The Loc-slope derived from localized muscle exercise was significantly correlated with the Sys-slope, the peak $\dot{V}_{O_2}$, and the AT in patients with CHF (Fig. 8).

Conclusions

These results suggest that impaired muscle metabolism associated with early metabolic limitation determines exercise capacity during maximal sys-

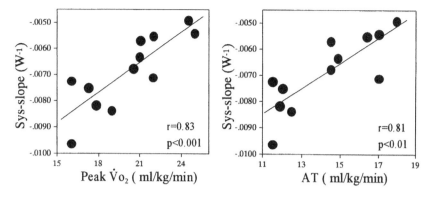

Figure 7. Significant correlations between muscle metabolic capacity evaluated as Sys-slope (PCr decrease to power output at the end of exercise) and the peak O_2 uptake (peak $\dot{V}O_2$) and the anaerobic threshold (AT). From Okita et al. Skeletal muscle metabolism limits exercise capacity in patients with chronic heart failure. Circulation 1998;98:1886-1891. Lippincott Williams & Wilkins.©

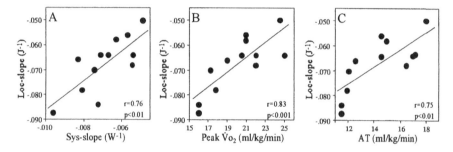

Figure 8. A. Relationship between the metabolic capacity during maximal systemic (Sys-slope) and local exercise (Loc-slope; the slope of the PCr decrease in relation to increases in the workload) in patients with chronic heart failure (CHF). **B.** Relationship between the peak $\dot{V}O_2$ and the Loc-slope in patients with CHF. **C.** Relationship between the anaerobic threshold (AT) and the Loc-slope in patients with CHF. From Okita et al. Skeletal muscle metabolism limits exercise capacity in patients with chronic heart failure. Circulation 1998;98:1886-1891. Lippincott Williams & Wilkins.©

temic exercise in patients with CHF. The intrinsic metabolic capacity during local exercise was significantly correlated with the metabolic capacity during systemic exercise and with the exercise capacity. The present studies suggest that exercise tolerance is governed largely by peripheral muscles. Factors affecting muscle metabolism, such as muscle intrinsic abnormalities, muscle mass, and muscle perfusion, may determine the exercise capacity in patients with CHF.

Previous studies have shown that an acute improvement in hemodynamics does not lead to an acute improvement in exercise tolerance in patients with CHF.[22] The explanation for this observation may be that an improvement in exercise tolerance requires an improvement in skeletal muscle metabolism. In fact, recent studies have demonstrated that exercise training can improve exercise tolerance, largely via peripheral adaptations in the absence of improvements to the central hemodynamic function.[23,24] We suggest that in most patients with CHF, skeletal muscle dysfunction may predominate over circulatory dysfunction. Thus, skeletal muscle training may improve exercise tolerance to the level that matches the circulatory capacity. And, if circulatory dysfunction is predominant, circulatory improvement may immediately improve exercise capacity by improving muscle perfusion.

Localized Skeletal Muscle Training

Can impaired skeletal muscle metabolism be improved by training without an improvement in cardiovascular performance? To determine an answer, we performed localized skeletal muscle training in patients with CHF.

Methods

Seven patients with CHF caused by idiopathic dilated cardiomyopathy were recruited into our training program.[25] The patients' mean age was 57 years, mean height was 167 cm, and mean weight was 69 kg. Six were in Class II of the New York Heart Association rankings for CHF, and the other patient was in Class III. All patients were taking digitalis, 5 were taking angiotensin-converting enzyme inhibitors, and 4 were taking beta-blockers. Pharmacological treatment was not altered for 3 months before and during the study. We contrived the training equipment for the right calf. The training protocol consisted of 1 set of right calf plantar flexion for 6 minutes. The workload was first set at 5 kg and was gradually increased up to 30 kg according to the subject's performance. Each patient did 4 sets of training a day, 5 to 7 days a week. Training was continued for 8 weeks. We evaluated the effects of training on muscle metabolism by having subjects do 6 minutes of plantar flexion at the submaximal workload (70% of the maximal work rate). The workload was determined according to the plantar flexion work capacity of the first incremental plantar flexion exercise test of each patient. We also measured muscle blood flow during plantar flexion by impedance plethysmography, and we evaluated systemic exercise tolerance with an upright bicycle ergometer. Comparisons were performed between post training and 8 weeks of detraining.

Results

Figure 9 shows the general effects of the plantar flexion training. Exertional fatigue was lessened with the training, and the MCA of the calf and the maximal voluntary contraction increased. Figure 10 shows the effect of training on muscle metabolism during exercise. There was a significant improvement in muscle metabolism during the training phase compared with the detraining phase. During 6 minutes of plantar flexion at the matched

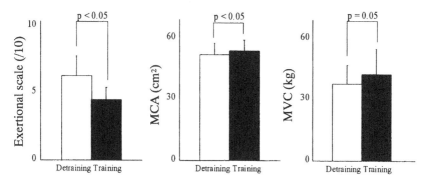

Figure 9. General effects of the exercise training of this study. Exertional scale (10-point scale of Borg); MCA = maximal cross-sectional area; MVC = maximal voluntary contraction. Open column = detraining phase; solid column = training phase.

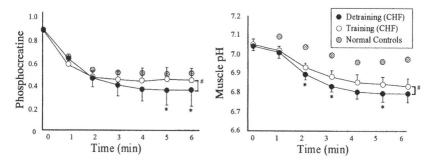

Figure 10. Significant training effect on muscle phosphocreatine depletion and muscle pH decrease during 6 minutes of plantar flexion at a constant workload. *p<0.05, #p<0.05 by analysis of variance versus training phase.

workload, both PCr and muscle pH were less decreased during the training phase than during the detraining phase. There was no significant change in calf blood flow between the training and detraining phases (rest 2.5±0.4 vs. 2.7±0.4, ns; exercise 27.6±2.4 vs. 29.8±2.7 mL/100 mL/min, ns, training, detraining, respectively).[25] Systemic exercise performance (peak $\dot{V}O_2$) was not changed significantly by this training (23.4±2.2 vs. 22.1±1.7 mL/kg/min, ns, training, detraining, respectively).

Conclusions

Impaired skeletal muscle metabolism during exercise was partly improved by the training, which might not have had any effect on cardiovascular capacity. The exertional symptoms that normally occur during exercise may also be improved by this training. There may be a specific muscle abnormality that is not related to muscle perfusion in patients with CHF. This type of training puts little stress on the cardiovascular system and can be performed safely; however, some problems remain. Although the training was continued for 8 weeks, muscle metabolism was not improved to a normal level. It is unknown if this type of training can improve a patient's prognosis as well as quality of life.

Summary

In the three studies reported in this chapter, we emphasize the important role of skeletal muscle metabolism during exercise in patients with CHF. Possible mechanisms for impaired muscle metabolism may be muscle atrophy, decreased aerobic enzyme activity, reduced mitochondrial volume, and fiber type alteration. Moreover, beyond the muscle, peripheral endothelial function, increased sympathetic nerve activity, and cardiac function might also be potential contributors. Since impaired muscle metabolism is observed during low levels of small muscle exercise, cardiac performance may not be a major reason for the impairment. One of the main mechanisms may be muscle deconditioning resulting from impaired cardiac performance. However, neither our group nor other researchers could not normalize the muscle metabolism even during localized muscle exercise by exercise training. This indicates that the important systemic factors may significantly affect the muscle metabolism.

Acknowledgment: I would like to thank the patients who participated in our studies. And I would also like to acknowledge my coworkers.

References

1. Lipkin DP, Jones DA, Round JM, Poole-Wilson PA. Abnormalities of skeletal muscle in patients with chronic heart failure. Int J Cardiol 1988;18:187-195.
2. Massie BM, Conway M, Rajagopalan B, et al. Skeletal muscle metabolism during exercise under ischemic conditions in congestive heart failure: evidence for abnormalities unrelated to blood flow. Circulation 1988;78:320-326.
3. Mancini DM, Ferraro N, Tuchler M, Chance B, Wilson JR. Detection of abnormal calf muscle metabolism in patients with heart failure using phosphorus-31 nuclear magnetic resonance. Am J Cardiol 1988;62:1234-1240.
4. Mancini DM, Coyle E, Coggan A, et al. Contribution of intrinsic skeletal muscle changes to ^{31}P NMR skeletal muscle metabolic abnormalities in patients with chronic heart failure. Circulation 1989;80:1338-1346.
5. Sullivan MJ, Green HJ, Cobb FR. Skeletal muscle biochemistry and histology in ambulatory patients with long-term heart failure. Circulation 1990;81:518-527.
6. Sullivan MJ, Green HJ, Cobb FR. Altered skeletal muscle metabolic response to exercise in chronic heart failure. Circulation 1991;84:1597-1607.
7. Mancini DM, Walter G, Reichek N, et al. Contribution of skeletal muscle atrophy to exercise intolerance and altered muscle metabolism in heart failure. Circulation 1992;85:1364-1373.
8. Drexler H, Reide U, Münzel T, König H, Just H. Alterations of skeletal muscle in chronic heart failure. Circulation 1992;85:1751-1759.

9. Minotti JR, Pillay P, Oka R, Wells L, Christoph I, Massie BM. Skeletal muscle size: relationship to muscle function in heart failure. J Appl Physiol 1993;75:373-381.

10. Chati Z, Zannad F, Robin-Lherbier B, et al. Contribution of specific skeletal muscle metabolic abnormalities to limitation of exercise capacity in patients with chronic heart failure: a phosphorus-31 nuclear magnetic resonance study. Am Heart J 1994;128:781-792.

11. Massie BM, Simonini A, Sahgal P, Wells L, Dudley GA. Relation of systemic and local muscle exercise capacity to skeletal characteristics in men with congestive heart failure. J Am Coll Cardiol 1996;27:104-145.

12. Okita K, Yonezawa K, Nishijima H, et al. Skeletal muscle metabolism limits exercise capacity in patients with chronic heart failure. Circulation 1998;98:1886-1891.

13. Hanada A, Okita K, Yonezawa K, et al. Dissociation between muscle metabolism and oxygen kinetics in patients with chronic heart failure. Heart 2000;83:161-166.

14. Okita K, Yonezawa K, Nishijima H, et al. Muscle high-energy metabolites and metabolic capacity in patients with heart failure. Med Sci Sport Exerc 2001;33:442-448.

15. Nishida M, Nishijima H, Yonezawa K, et al. Phosphorus-31 magnetic resonance spectroscopy of forearm flexor muscles in student rowers using an exercise protocol adjusted for differences in cross-sectional muscle area. Eur J Appl Physiol 1992;64:528-533.

16. Taylor DJ, Bore PJ, Styles P, Gadian DG, Radda GK. Bioenergetics of intact human muscle: a ^{31}P nuclear magnetic resonance study. Mol Biol Med 1983;1:77-94.

17. Dawson MJ, Gadian DG, Wilkie DR. Contraction and recovery of living muscles studies by ^{31}P nuclear magnetic resonance. J Physiol 1977;267:703-735.

18. Jeneson JA, Taylor JS, Vigneron DB, et al. ^{1}H MR imaging of anatomical compartments within the finger flexor muscles of human forearm. Magn Reson Med 1990;15:481-496.

19. Wasserman K, Whipp BJ, Koyal SN, Beaver WL. Anaerobic threshold and respiratory gas exchange during exercise. J Appl Physiol 1972;33:351-356.

20. Harris RC, Edwards RH, Hultman E, Nordesjö L-O, Nylind B, Sahlin K. The time course of phosphorylcreatine resynthesis during recovery of the quadriceps muscle in man. Pflugers Arch 1976;367:137-142.

21. Okita K, Nishijima H, Yonezawa K, et al. Skeletal muscle metabolism in maximal bicycle and treadmill exercise distinguished by using in-vivo metabolic freeze method and phosphorus-31 magnetic resonance spectroscopy in normal men. Am J Cardiol 1998;81:106-109.

22. Maskin CS, Forman R, Sonnenblick EH, Frishman WH, LeJemtel TH. Failure of dobutamine to increase exercise capacity despite hemodynamic improvement in severe chronic heart failure. Am J Cardiol 1983;51:177-182.

23. Minotti JR, Johonson EC, Hudson TL, et al. Training-induced skeletal muscle adaptations are independent of systemic adaptations. J Appl Physiol 1990;68:289-294.

24. Belardinelli R, Georgiou D, Scocco V, Barstow TJ, Purcaro A. Low intensity exercise training in patients with chronic heart failure. J Am Coll Cardiol 1995;26:975-982.

25. Ohtsubo M, Yonezawa K, Nishijima H, et al. Metabolic abnormality of calf skeletal muscle is improved by localized muscle training without changes in blood flow in chronic heart failure. Heart 1997;78:437-443.

Section 2

Grading Heart Failure and Predicting Survival

3

Predicting Survival in Heart Failure:

Exercise-Based Prognosticating Algorithms

Donna Mancini, MD

Measurement of O_2 uptake ($\dot{V}O_2$) in patients with chronic heart failure (CHF) was first described by Weber et al.[1] as a noninvasive method for characterizing cardiac reserve and functional status in these patients. Its value as a prognostic marker in heart failure became apparent shortly thereafter. Szlachcic et al.[2] described a 77% 1-year mortality rate for patients with a $\dot{V}O_2$ <10 mL/kg/min in a group of 27 patients with CHF versus a 21% mortality rate for those with a $\dot{V}O_2$ of 10 to 18 mL/kg/min. Likoff et al.[3] described a 36% mortality rate in 201 patients with heart failure with a $\dot{V}O_2$ <13 mL/kg/min compared with 15% when $\dot{V}O_2$ exceeded 13 mL/kg/min. Analysis of the exercise data from the original Veterans Administration Heart Failure Trial (VHeFT) also demonstrated that $\dot{V}O_2$ was an independent prognostic indicator[4] for mortality. However, it was not until measurement of $\dot{V}O_2$ was applied to the cardiac transplant candidate selection process that the clinical use of this parameter became widespread.

The first study to investigate whether peak exercise $\dot{V}O_2$ could help to optimally time cardiac transplant was performed at the University of Pennsylvania. From October 1986 to December 1989, all ambulatory patients referred for cardiac transplantation underwent cardiopulmonary testing.[5] A total of 116 patients were divided into three groups based on the results of their stress tests. Group 1 consisted of patients with a peak $\dot{V}O_2$ below 14 mL/kg/min who were accepted as transplant candidates (n=35). Group 2 were patients with a peak $\dot{V}O_2$ >14 mL/kg/min who had transplant deferred

From Wasserman K (ed): *Cardiopulmonary Exercise Testing and Cardiovascular Health.* Armonk, NY: Futura Publishing Company, Inc.; © 2002.

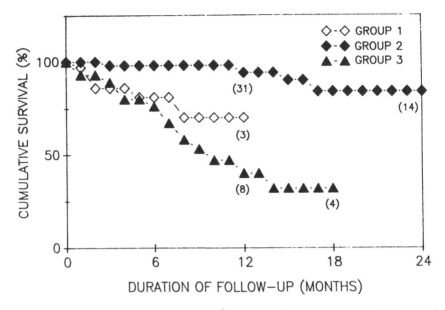

Figure 1. Survival curves for patients with V̇O₂ >14 mL/kg/min (group 2) and those with V̇O₂ <14 mL/kg/min (groups 1 and 3). From Mancini et al.,[5] with permission.

(n=52), and group 3 comprised patients with a peak $\dot{V}_{O_2}$ <14 mL/kg/min but with a significant comorbidity which precluded transplant (n=27). Age, left ventricular ejection fraction, and resting hemodynamic parameters were similar among the groups. As depicted in Figure 1, 1-year survival was 94% in the patient group with a $\dot{V}_{O_2}$ >14 mL/kg/min. Accepted transplant candidates with a $\dot{V}_{O_2}$ <14 mL/kg/min had a 1-year survival of 70%, whereas those patients with a significant comorbidity and reduced $\dot{V}_{O_2}$ had a 1-year survival of 47%. Patients accepted for transplant had a falsely elevated survival, as all transplants were treated as a censored observation. If urgent transplant was counted as death, 1-year survival fell to 48%. Using this approach, candidates were identified in whom cardiac transplant could be safely deferred. Subsequent to this study, the application of cardiopulmonary stress testing for the selection of potential transplant candidates has gained widespread acceptance in the US. Measurement of $\dot{V}_{O_2}$ is now considered a critical branch point in typical algorithms for selection of ambulatory cardiac transplant candidates.[6]

Percent of Predicted Peak V̇O₂

Age, gender, muscle mass, and conditioning status can impact on peak $\dot{V}_{O_2}$. The multiple factors that affect peak exercise capacity may explain why some patients with CHF and a peak $\dot{V}_{O_2}$ <14 mL/kg/min have a favorable prognosis even when transplant is deferred. Accordingly, we investigated whether percent of predicted peak $\dot{V}O_2$ would yield better risk stratification than the absolute value.[7] Peak $\dot{V}O_2$ was measured in 272 patients with advanced CHF who were referred for transplant evaluation. Predicted peak $\dot{V}O_2$ was then calculated for each patient using the Astrand and Wasserman equations. Patients were then divided into three groups: those with a peak $\dot{V}O_2$ <10 mL/kg/min, those with $\dot{V}O_2$ 10 to 14 mL/kg/min, and those with $\dot{V}O_2$ > 14 mL/kg/min. Strata for percent predicted peak $\dot{V}O_2$ were determined by cut points that would yield strata of similar size to the above groups. Survival curves for patients stratified by absolute and percent peak $\dot{V}O_2$ were very similar. Receiver operating curves were constructed for absolute peak $\dot{V}O_2$ normalized for body weight and percentage of predicted maximal $\dot{V}O_2$. The area under the curves was roughly equal; therefore, normalization of peak exercise $\dot{V}O_2$ for predicted values added minimal prognostic information.

A similar study of the application of percent predicted $\dot{V}O_2$ as a prognostic marker was conducted by Stelken et al.[8] This study was a retrospective review of 181 patients who were referred to their heart failure center. Clinical, hemodynamic, and coronary angiographic data were recorded and all patients underwent symptom-limited cardiopulmonary exercise. The actuarial 1- and 2-year survival of the 89 patients who achieved ≤50% predicted peak $\dot{V}O_2$ was 74% and 43%, respectively, compared to 98% and 90% in the 92 who achieved >50% predicted peak $\dot{V}O_2$ (p=0.001). Multivariate analysis selected ≤50% predicted peak $\dot{V}O_2$ as the most significant predictor of cardiac death (p=0.007). Based on these findings, the authors concluded that patients who achieve >50% predicted peak $\dot{V}O_2$ have an excellent short-term prognosis when treated medically, and heart transplantation can thus be safely deferred in this population.

Peak $\dot{V}O_2$ is a continuous rather than a discrete variable, and differences in the above two studies may be explained by both investigators attempting to assign a threshold or cut-off value to determine transplant candidacy. Stratum-specific likelihood ratios can be used to identify threshold values. We therefore calculated stratum-specific likelihood ratios in 140 ambulatory patients referred for cardiac transplant evaluation.[9] The ratios progressively increased, the higher the peak $\dot{V}O_2$, without identification of a discrete cut point. Therefore, these stratum-specific likelihood ratios indicate that peak $\dot{V}O_2$ is a strong and continuous predictor of survival in this population without an absolute threshold.

Exercise Hemodynamic Measurements with $\dot{V}O_2$

In a further attempt to enhance the predictive power of peak exercise $\dot{V}O_2$, some investigators have coupled hemodynamic monitoring with $\dot{V}O_2$ measurements. Chomsky et al.[10] evaluated cardiopulmonary and hemodynamic exercise responses of 185 ambulatory patients with CHF and a mean peak $\dot{V}O_2$ of 12.9 mL/kg/min referred for transplant evaluation. In this study the authors used the following formula to define a normal cardiac output response to exercise: cardiac output = 5 × $\dot{V}O_2$ (L/min) + 3 L/min. Based on this formula, they divided the cohort into normal and reduced cardiac output groups. Multivariate analysis found that both a peak $\dot{V}O_2$ <10 mL/kg/min and a reduced cardiac output response to exercise as defined by the above equation were predictive of a poor 1-year survival. The major concern regarding this study is the derivation of the formula used to define a normal output response. Derived from the work of Higginbotham et al.,[11] this formula adapts hemodynamic data from younger normal subjects performing a different type of exercise (i.e., upright bicycle not treadmill exercise). Chomsky et al.[10] extrapolated these data into an area of the curve where there are minimal hard data, and further modified the curve by using an assumed mean body surface area of 1.8 m^2. Their multivariate analysis also did not include directly measured peak exercise hemodynamic values such as peak cardiac output, peak pulmonary capillary wedge pressure, etc. Whether a straightforward multivariate analysis using directly measured values would have yielded similar findings is unclear.

We also investigated whether exercise hemodynamic measurements could better identify patients at an increased risk, rather than peak $\dot{V}O_2$ alone.[12] Sixty-five patients underwent bicycle exercise with simultaneous metabolic and hemodynamic measurements. Peak $\dot{V}O_2$ was 12.1±3 mL/kg/min, pulmonary capillary wedge 31±11 mm Hg, cardiac output 7.6±2.2 L/min, cardiac index 3.8±1.3 L/min, and pulmonary artery oxyhemoglobin saturation 27±9%. A variety of hemodynamic variables were examined, including the relation between $\dot{V}O_2$ and pulmonary artery saturation via algebraic manipulation of the Fick equation. A $\dot{V}O_2$ intercept and slope of the $\dot{V}O_2$-pulmonary artery saturation relation were derived for each patient.

Of the 65 patients, 16 died or underwent urgent transplant. Results of multivariate analysis demonstrated that the only exercise variable predictive of survival was left ventricular stroke work and index. These results were consistent with those of Griffin et al.[13] who, using multiple logistic regression analysis, identified peak exercise stroke work index as the only exercise-derived hemodynamic predictor of mortality. More recently, Metra et al.[14] studied 219 consecutive patients with CHF. Bicycle cardiopulmonary stress testing with hemodynamic monitoring was performed. Mean follow-up was 19 months. By Cox multivariate analysis, peak exercise stroke work index was the most sensitive predictor of survival. This parameter, however, is highly dependent on the degree of mitral regurgitation. As mitral regurgitation was not directly measured in any of these studies, the accuracy of this finding is questionable. Therefore, it is difficult to advocate the widespread application of this particular variable.

Measurement of exercise hemodynamics does not appear to significantly improve risk stratification beyond that provided by direct measurement of $\dot{V}O_2$. Moreover, its potential benefit is outweighed by the increased complexity and expense of exercise hemodynamic testing.

To further stratify the high-risk group of patients with $\dot{V}O_2$ <14 mL/ kg/min, Osada et al.[15] performed multivariate analysis using all noninvasive exercise parameters measured during exercise testing. Cardiopulmonary exercise testing was performed in 500 patients with CHF referred for heart transplantation; 154 (31%) had a peak exercise $\dot{V}O_2$ ≤14 mL/kg/min. Multivariate analyses of exercise and cardiopulmonary variables (i.e., peak exercise heart rate, systolic blood pressure, respiratory exchange ratio, minute ventilation, peak $\dot{V}O_2$, percent predicted peak $\dot{V}O_2$, and anaerobic threshold) were performed to identify the 3-year prognostic risk. Peak systolic blood pressure <120 mm Hg (p=0.0005) and percent predicted peak $\dot{V}O_2$ ≤50% (p= 0.04) were significant prognostic variables in patients with a peak $\dot{V}O_2$ ≤14 mL/kg/min. Survival was 55% at 3 years for the 77 patients with a peak exercise $\dot{V}O_2$ ≤14 mL/kg/min and peak exercise systolic blood pressure <120 mm Hg versus an 83% survival rate in the 74 patients able to reach this exercise blood pressure (p=0.004).

Heart Failure Survival Score

Although powerful as an independent variable, selection and stratification of transplant candidates based solely on a simple dichotomization by peak $\dot{V}O_2$ is limited. Such an approach does not make efficient use of routinely obtained clinical measures of known prognostic significance such as left ventricular ejection fraction. Pretransplant risk stratification could be improved by developing a predictive model that incorporates multiple independent predictors of mortality. Most prior multivariate analyses have not developed threshold values or have been prospectively validated.[16-18]

We therefore developed a heart failure survival score from 467 ambulatory patients with severe CHF followed at two institutions from July 1986 to September 1994.[19] The model was developed on 268 patients at the hospital of the University of Pennsylvania who were followed from July 1986 to September 1993. It was validated on a group of 199 patients at Columbia Presbyterian Hospital from July 1993 to October 1995.

Eighty clinical variables on each patient derived from clinical history, physical exam, laboratory, exercise, and catheterization data were entered into the data set. Univariate survival analyses were performed using Kaplan-Meier analyses. Significant univariate factors were then analyzed with multivariate techniques. Variables were grouped and those prognostic factors felt to represent different aspects of CHF were incorporated into the model. In construction of the model, clinical judgment was used to guide the selection process. Variables that incorporated multiple aspects of the pathophysiology of heart failure were placed in the model.

Two models were constructed. One statistical model incorporated exclusively noninvasive parameters. The other included all measured variables derived from noninvasive as well as invasive tests. The model with the

_____ Table 1 _____

Calculation of the Heart Failure Survival Score
for a Patient with Coronary Artery Disease and Normal ECG

Clinical Characteristic	Value	Model Coefficient	Product
Ischemic cardiomyopathy	1	+0.6931	+0.6931
Resting heart rate	90	+0.0216	+1.9440
LVEF	17	-0.0464	-0.7888
Mean BP	80	-0.0255	-2.0400
IVCD	0	+0.6083	0
Peak $\dot{V}O_2$	16.2	-0.0546	-0.8845
Serum sodium	132	-0.0470	-6.2040

Prognostic score = |sum of the products| = 7.2802.
BP = blood pressure; IVCD= intraventricular conduction defect; LVEF= left ventricular ejection fraction; |. . .| = absolute value.

smallest number of variables that could most accurately predict survival was derived. The best model included 7 variables: presence or absence of coronary artery disease, resting heart rate, left ventricular ejection fraction, mean arterial blood pressure, presence or absence of intraventricular conduction defect on baseline electrocardiogram, peak $\dot{V}O_2$, and serum sodium. Beta coefficients were assigned from the Cox model with the hazard ratio and level of significance. The noninvasive model included parameters that estimated myocardial ischemia (ischemic cardiomyopathy), the degree of systolic dysfunction (left ventricular ejection fraction), the degree of activation of the renin-angiotensin system (serum sodium), activation of sympathetic nervous system (heart rate), the extent of myocardial fibrosis and injury (intraventricular conduction defect), and more integrative measures such as peak $\dot{V}O_2$ and mean arterial blood pressure. The invasive model included pulmonary capillary wedge in addition to the above variables. It performed similar to the noninvasive model. Therefore, to simplify its use in clinical practice, our emphasis has been on the use of the noninvasive model. Table 1 shows the calculation of a prognostic score for a typical transplant candidate. The value of the variable and the beta coefficient are multiplied and the products added. The absolute value of the sum represents the prognostic score. For noncontinuous variables, i.e., coronary artery disease or intraventricular conduction defect, their presence is assigned a value of 1 and their absence a value of zero.

Model discrimination was tested using receiver operating curves and censored c index. Threshold levels for the prognostic score were determined by stratum-specific likelihood ratios. Stratum-specific likelihood ratios revealed 3 distinct groups in the derivation data set. Those patients with excellent survival had prognostic scores above 8.1 whereas those patients at greatest risk had scores lower than 7.2. Similar survival curves could be generated in the Columbia validation sample. Thus, the application of this statistical model, which incorporates several prognostic factors, should help to more effectively risk stratify patients. In a recent publication by Deng et al.,[20] application of the heart failure survival score in 889 adult patients listed for transplant correctly identified high-risk patients.

Heart failure is a dynamic process. Cardiac transplant evaluation collects prognostic variables at one point in this disease process. Accordingly, the importance of reevaluation of these candidates has been emphasized. Stevenson et al.[21] initially reported improved survival for those patients waiting for cardiac transplant for more than 6 months. They concluded that these patients derive less benefit from cardiac transplantation the longer they wait for the procedure. However, for most patients CHF is a progressive disease. These conclusions are therefore circumspect. Analysis of a similar cohort of patients who are listed for cardiac transplantation, after full optimization of medical therapy, showed continued poor survival in those candidates without transplant compared to those with cardiac transplantation.[22]

Serial assessment of continued transplant eligibility has included repeated measures of peak $\dot{V}O_2$.[23,24] Patients who respond to alteration of medical therapy, and have objective evidence of improvement with a significant increase in peak $\dot{V}O_2$, may be able to have their transplant deferred as 1- to 2-year survival is comparable to post-transplant survival.

Summary

Peak $\dot{V}O_2$ is a powerful predictor for short-term prognosis in patients with CHF. It is a valuable clinical tool for identifying potential transplant candidates. Serial assessment of exercise capacity provides useful clinical information for long-term care of these patients.

References

1. Weber K, Kinasewitz G, Janicki J, Fishman A. Oxygen utilization and ventilation during exercise in patients with chronic congestive heart failure. Circulation 1982;65:1213-1223.

2. Szlachcic J, Massie B, Kramer B, Topic N, Tubau J. Correlates and prognostic implication of exercise capacity in chronic congestive heart failure. Am J Cardiol 1985;55:1037-1042.

3. Likoff MJ, Chandler SL, Kay HR. Clinical determinants of mortality in chronic congestive heart failure secondary to idiopathic dilated or to ischemic cardiomyopathy. Am J Cardiol 1987;59:634-638.

4. Cohn J, Johnson G, Shabetai R, et al., for the V-Heft VA Cooperative Studies Group. Ejection fraction, peak exercise oxygen consumption, cardiothoracic ratio, ventricular arrhythmias, and plasma norepinephrine as determinants of prognosis in heart failure. Circulation 1993;87:VI5-VI16.

5. Mancini DM, Eisen H, Kussmaul W, Mull R, Edmunds LH, Wilson JR. Value of peak exercise oxygen consumption for optimal timing of cardiac transplantation in ambulatory patients with heart failure. Circulation 1991;83:778-786.

6. Costanzo M, Augustine S, Bourge R, et al. Selection and treatment of candidates for heart transplantation. Circulation 1995;92:3593-3612.

7. Aaronson KD, Mancini DM. Is percentage of predicted maximal exercise oxygen consumption a better predictor of survival than peak exercise oxygen consumption for patients with severe heart failure? J Heart Lung Transplant 1995;14: 981-989.

8. Stelken AM, Younis LT, Jennison SH, et al. Prognostic value of cardiopulmonary exercise testing using percent achieved of predicted peak oxygen uptake for patients with ischemic and dilated cardiomyopathy. J Am Coll Cardiol 1996; 27:345-352.

9. Aaronson K, Chen T, Mancini D. Demonstration of the continuous nature of peak $\dot{V}O_2$ for predicting survival in ambulatory patients evaluated for transplant. J Heart Lung Transplant 1996;15:S66.

10. Chomsky DB, Lange CC, Rayos GH, et al. Hemodynamic exercise testing: a valuable tool in the selection of cardiac transplantation candidates. Circulation 1996;94:3176-3183.

11. Higginbotham MB, Morris KG, Williams RS, McHale PA, Coleman RE, Cobb FR. Regulation of stroke volume during submaximal and maximal upright exercise in normal man. Circ Res 1986;58:281-291.

12. Mancini D, Katz S, Donchez L, Aaronson K. Coupling of hemodynamic measurements with oxygen consumption during exercise does not improve risk stratification in patients with heart failure. Circulation 1996;94:2492-2496.

13. Griffin B, Shah P, Ferguson J, Rubin S. Incremental prognostic value of exercise hemodynamic variables in chronic congestive heart failure secondary to coronary artery disease or to dilated cardiomyopathy. Am J Cardiol 1991;67:848-853.

14. Metra M, Faggiano P, D'Aloia A, et al. Use of cardiopulmonary exercise testing with hemodynamic monitoring in the prognostic assessment of ambulatory patients with congestive heart failure. J Am Coll Cardiol 1999;33:943-950.

15. Osada N, Chaitman BR, Miller LW, et al. Cardiopulmonary exercise testing identifies low risk patients with heart failure and severely impaired exercise capacity considered for heart transplantation. J Am Coll Cardiol 1998;31:577-582.

16. Unverferth D, Magorien R, Moeschberger M, Baker P, Fetters J, Leier C. Factors influencing the one-year mortality of dilated cardiomyopathy. Am J Cardiol 1984;54:147-152.

17. Lee W, Packer M. Prognostic importance of serum sodium concentration and its modification by converting-enzyme inhibition in patients with severe chronic heart failure. Circulation 1986;73:257-267.

18. Wilson J, Schwartz J, Sutton M, et al. Prognosis in severe heart failure: relation to hemodynamic measurements and ventricular ectopic activity. J Am Coll Cardiol 1983;2:403-410.

19. Aaronson K, Schwartz JS, Chen T, Wong K, Goin J, Mancini D. Development and prospective validation of a clinical index to predict survival in ambulatory patients referred for cardiac transplant evaluation. Circulation 1997;95:2660-2667.

20. Deng M, De Meester J, Smits J, Heinecke J, Scheld H. Effect of receiving a heart transplant: analysis of a national cohort entered on to a waiting list stratified by heart failure severity. Br Med J 2000;321:540-545.

21. Stevenson WG, Stevenson LW, Middlekauff HR, et al. Improving survival for patients with advanced heart failure: a study of 737 consecutive patients. J Am Coll Cardiol 1995;26:1417-1423.

22. Aaronson K, Bowers J, Chen T, Mancini D. Mortality remains high for outpatient transplant candidates with prolonged (>6 months) waiting list time. J Am Coll Cardiol 1999;33:1189-1195.

23. Stevenson L, Steimle A, Fonarow G, et al. Improvement in exercise capacity of candidates awaiting heart transplantation. J Am Coll Cardiol 1995;25:163-170.

24. Aaronson K, Bowers J, Gonzalez J, Mancini D. Heart failure survival model predicts survival when applied serially at subsequent reevaluation. J Heart Lung Transplant 1997;17:82A.

4

Grading Heart Failure and Predicting Survival:

Slope of $\dot{V}_E$ versus $\dot{V}_{CO_2}$

Andrew J.S. Coats, MA, DM

Chronic heart failure (CHF) is a common condition with a poor prognosis. It is characteristically associated with poor exercise tolerance and debilitating symptoms despite optimal modern therapy. Optimization of management and selection for special treatments depends on a reliable system for identifying high-risk patients. For decades clinicians have attempted to find a reliable marker for prognosis in patients with CHF. Ideally, the marker should be widely applicable, associated with disease severity, reproducible, and indicative of response to therapy. Much attention has recently been focused on parameters derived from cardiopulmonary exercise testing. Of the many parameters that can be obtained from an analysis of respiratory gases during incremental exercise, the relationship between minute ventilation and the rate of CO_2 elimination at the mouth (the $\dot{V}_E$ vs. $\dot{V}_{CO_2}$ slope) has achieved strong attention as being reliable, reproducible, strongly related to mortality, and easy to acquire in the clinical evaluation of a patient. While we do not fully understand the pathophysiological mechanisms underlying the cause of the characteristically high $\dot{V}_E$ vs. $\dot{V}_{CO_2}$ slope of CHF, many studies have attested to its reliable prognostic value. The causes that have been suggested as contributing to the elevated slope in CHF include ventilation/perfusion (V/Q) mismatch, non-CO_2 stimuli to ventilation, impaired pulmonary blood flow, and pulmonary vasoconstriction. This chapter describes the data evaluating the prognostic utility of the $\dot{V}_E$ vs. $\dot{V}_{CO_2}$ slope

Professor Coats is supported by the Viscount Royston Trust, the British Heart Foundation, the Clinical Research Committee of the Royal Brompton Hospital, and the Asmarley Trust.

From Wasserman K (ed): *Cardiopulmonary Exercise Testing and Cardiovascular Health.* Armonk, NY: Futura Publishing Company, Inc.; © 2002.

and attempts to summarize some of the studies that have investigated the clinical associates, treatment interventions, and pathophysiological mechanisms underlying this cardiopulmonary response in CHF patients.

Foremost among the symptoms of CHF is dyspnea at low exercise workloads and impaired exercise capacity. The severity of symptomatic exercise limitation varies among patients, and this appears to bear little relationship to the extent of the left ventricular systolic dysfunction measured at rest, or to markers of hemodynamic disturbance. Study of cardiopulmonary responses to progressive exercise has helped us better understand the physiological processes underlying the generation of symptoms in this condition. It has also identified parameters associated with disability and even poor prognosis in CHF. Among these changes is an increase in the slope of the relationship between minute ventilation ($\dot{V}E$) and the rate of CO_2 output ($\dot{V}CO_2$).[1] This slope has been found to correlate with the severity of symptoms, the perception of dyspnea, a poor prognosis, and objective limitation of exercise as assessed by peak O_2 uptake (peak $\dot{V}O_2$).[2,3]

The slope of the relationship between $\dot{V}E$ and $\dot{V}CO_2$ during progressive exercise is approximately linear for most subjects at least until near maximal exercise. There are deviations from linearity in more severe heart failure cases.[4] The linear component of the relationship (slope) is increased in heart failure. Possible causes include V/Q mismatch within the lung causing excessive but noncontributory (dead space) ventilation,[5] and/or increased alveolar ventilation leading to hypocapnia (decreased arterial PCO_2), or a combination of the two. As Johnson[6] recently editorialized in *Circulation*, "A high $\dot{V}E/CO_2$ ratio has 2 possible sources: (1) increased ventilation, which is required to overcome a large dead space to maintain a normal arterial CO_2 tension ($PaCO_2$), or (2) increased central drive to ventilation, which drives the $PaCO_2$ below what is normally expected." The relative contributions of these two mechanisms have long been argued.[7] However, because blood gases remain relatively normal in heart failure patients during exercise, the ventilatory increase relative to increase in $\dot{V}CO_2$ has long been thought to be due to an increase in physiological dead space/tidal volume ratio (VD/VT), since the only determinants of $\dot{V}E$ are $\dot{V}CO_2$, $PaCO_2$, and VD/VT, as shown in the following alveolar ventilation equation:

$$\dot{V}E = 863 \ \dot{V}CO_2/([PaCO_2 \ (1- \ VD/VT)]$$

where 863 is a constant for conversion of fractional concentration of PCO_2 to partial pressure and water vapor corrections for conversions from ambient temperature and pressure, saturated with water vapor, to $\dot{V}CO_2$ as standard temperature and pressure dry and $\dot{V}E$ as body temperature pressure saturated. This of course pertains to steady state conditions, and application of this equation during progressive exercise in CHF patients when steady state conditions may not apply might be misleading. Increasing ventilation may be associated with delays in CO_2 delivery to the lungs, and may be associated with transients in CO_2 stores in venous blood.

The ergoreflex system senses the metabolic state of exercising skeletal muscle and reflexly increases ventilation. It is sensed by small work-sensitive afferents and its afferent limb is carried by small myelinated or unmyelinated nerve fibers. Recent studies suggest that an overactivity of these fibers and the resultant reflex account for the abnormal ventilatory responses described in CHF in both arm[8] and leg exercise.[9] The chemoreceptor system controlling ventilation may also be overactive. We recently described augmentation of peripheral hypoxic and central CO_2 sensitivity in CHF patients.[10] Andreas et al.[11] described that the increased ventilatory response to CO_2 correlates impressively with the $\dot{V}$E vs. $\dot{V}$CO$_2$ slope. The hypercapnic ventilatory response was measured at rest using the rebreathing method in 31 patients with CHF and in 25 controls. $\dot{V}$E vs. $\dot{V}$CO$_2$ slope during exercise was positively correlated to the hypercapnic ventilatory response (r=0.70; p<0.00001). The authors concluded that different afferents to the respiratory center, such as central command or muscle ergoreflex, may play a role in modulating ventilation during exercise. These altered ventilatory control reflexes could explain part of the heightened ventilatory responses acting in concert with V/Q mismatch. The cause of the heightened chemosensitivity itself remains undetermined, but it is possible that there is a direct interaction between the ergoreflex and chemoreflex systems. We have shown in a series of 173 CHF patients that the clinical features associated with an elevated $\dot{V}$E vs. $\dot{V}$CO$_2$ slope include increased age (62.2 vs. 57.3 years, p=0.005), New York Heart Association (NYHA) functional class (2.9 vs. 2.1, p<0.001), left ventricular ejection fraction (24.7 vs. 31.9%, p=0.0016), reduced peak $\dot{V}$O$_2$ (14.9 vs. 21.7 mL/kg/min, p<0.0001), and increased radiographic cardiothoracic ratio (0.58 vs. 0.55, p=0.002).[12] Because some authors have argued that PaCO$_2$ remains relatively unchanged or decreases only slightly at higher work rates when lactic acidosis supervenes,[13] they claim that the elevated $\dot{V}$E vs. $\dot{V}$CO$_2$ slope must be mainly due to the increase in VD/VT. A recent reanalysis of individual patient data from an earlier publication by Franciosa et al.[14] showed convincingly, however, that although the mean PaCO$_2$ (35±7 mm Hg) was the same at rest and peak exercise, individual patient blood gas and hemodynamic data showed some CHF patients with lowered PaCO$_2$ values on exercise. This allowed a more comprehensive analysis.[6] Both the $\dot{V}$E vs. $\dot{V}$CO$_2$ and VD/VT ratios can be calculated at peak exercise from the tabulated data and plotted with respect to PaCO$_2$. This yielded a highly significant inverse correlation between $\dot{V}$E vs. $\dot{V}$CO$_2$ and PaCO$_2$ that supports the hypothesis presented by Ponikowski et al. stating that increased sensitivity of ventilatory control is important in some patients in causing an elevated slope.[6] A highly significant, direct correlation between $\dot{V}$E vs. $\dot{V}$CO$_2$ and the VD/VT ratio was also seen, confirming an uneven distribution of ventilation with respect to perfusion in the lung. Thus, the PaCO$_2$ was seen to be driven to low levels during peak exercise in CHF, despite inefficient gas exchange from a high V_D/V_T ratio.[6]

Ventilatory Response to Exercise in CHF

At between 85% and 95% of peak $\dot{V}O_2$ in patients with CHF, a point in exercise is reached where there is an excessive release of CO_2 for the rate of $\dot{V}O_2$ resulting from a limitation in the rate of delivery of O_2 that leads to the onset of anaerobic muscular metabolism with lactate production. This produces arterial acidosis and directly stimulates the chemoreceptors to increase ventilation further. This point is called the anaerobic threshold (AT), although whether it truly represents a distinct transition point has been debated.

In most normal subjects, exercise is limited by cardiac reserve with lung function rarely being the limiting factor. In nonedematous stable and optimally treated patients with CHF, submaximal exercise and the hemodynamic response accompanying it may be remarkably normal, with only an increase in nonessential vascular bed vasoconstrictor drive providing evidence of a limited cardiac reserve. There is, however, despite preservation of arterial gas concentrations, an exaggerated ventilatory response even at low-level exercise. Most patients with CHF fail to achieve their peak $\dot{V}O_2$, and it has been shown that, in contrast to normal subjects, the addition of arm exercise to a patient already performing maximal leg exercise leads to a further increase in the rate of $\dot{V}O_2$.[13] This shows that O_2 delivery, and by extrapolation cardiac output, may not be maximal during maximal leg exercise test in the CHF patients. The true limiting factor to exercise appears to reside in the inadequate peripheral use of O_2 for regeneration of high-energy phosphate (adenosine triphosphate), because of either a defect in the peripheral vasculature or abnormality of the bioenergetic processes in the skeletal muscle.

Even below the AT there is an exaggerated ventilatory response with reference to CO_2 production in most patients with CHF. The response is near linear but the slope is significantly increased. The mechanisms underlying this increased ventilatory response remain uncertain. In one multicenter report on 130 patients with CHF and 52 normal controls,[15] spirometric and breath-by-breath gas exchange measurements were made during rest and increasing cycle exercise in an effort to determine the features associated with this response. Arterial blood was sampled for measurement of pH, $PaCO_2$, PaO_2, and lactate during exercise in 85 patients. Patients with more severe CHF had a higher respiratory rate and a smaller tidal volume (V_T) at a given $\dot{V}E$. The V_D/V_T ratio increased inversely with peak $\dot{V}O_2/kg$. While the $PaCO_2$ response was normal, $P_{ET}CO_2$ was reduced and $PaCO_2 - P_{ET}CO_2$ was increased as peak $\dot{V}O_2$ decreased. In contrast, the difference between alveolar and arterial PO_2 was normal, on average, at peak $\dot{V}O_2$ regardless of the level of impairment. The authors concluded that the increase in $\dot{V}E$ seen in the CHF patients was likely to be caused by the increase in VD/VT resulting from high V/Q mismatching, an increase in $\dot{V}CO_2$ relative to $\dot{V}O_2$ resulting from HCO_3^- buffering of lactic acid, and a decrease in $PaCO_2$ due to tight regulation of arterial pH. With regard to the excessive $\dot{V}E$ in CHF patients, the increases in VD/VT and $\dot{V}CO_2$ relative to $\dot{V}O_2$ appeared to be more important as the patients were more limited. Regional hypoperfusion but not hypoventilation typifies lung gas exchange in CHF. This and other mechanisms might account for the restrictive changes leading to exercise tachypnea in CHF patients.

While fitting the data, these explanations require that a primary reduction in lung perfusion or mismatch in perfusion to ventilation occurs. This having been sensed, ventilation increases appropriately to the increase in CO_2 generated from aerobic metabolism and the HCO_3^- buffering of lactic acid, albeit with reduced efficiency (high slope of $\dot{V}E$ vs. $\dot{V}CO_2$) because of the high VD/VT. Alveolar ventilation, however, must by this hypothesis be appropriate for the increased $\dot{V}CO_2$ as dictated by the normal $PaCO_2$. The increase in pulmonary vascular resistance associated with the loss of capillary bed and reflected in the increase in VD/VT is consistent with the findings that exercise limitation shows a significantly better correlation with measures of right ventricular function than with left ventricular function.[16]

Chauhan et al.[17] found that in 7 patients with stable CHF the addition of extra dead space did not significantly alter peak $\dot{V}O_2$, workload, heart rate, or exercise duration, which were not significantly different between the added dead space and control tests. The breathing pattern was significantly deeper and slower at matched levels of ventilation during exercise with added dead space, in contrast to what is seen in CHF patients without added dead space. A primary increase in relative dead space would therefore not seem likely to be the predominant cause of the rapid, shallow ventilation and reduced exercise tolerance (that is tightly linked to increased $\dot{V}E$ vs. $\dot{V}CO_2$ slope) of CHF patients. Thus, although increased dead space seems to inevitably be associated with an increase in the $\dot{V}E$ vs. $\dot{V}CO_2$ slope, attempts to further increase VD do not mimic the abnormalities characteristic of CHF.

Measurements of V/Q Matching in the Lungs

An obligate result of V/Q mismatch is an increase in VD/VT, because dead space ventilation not only includes the anatomical dead space of the lungs but also has added alveolar dead space (underperfused alveolar units). Wada and colleagues,[18] using scintigraphic count ratio (technetium 99m macroaggregated albumin) of upper to lower lung fields in 23 patients with CHF and 9 age-matched normal subjects, found that blood flow was redistributed to the upper lung zones in those patients in whom the slope of $\dot{V}E$ vs. $\dot{V}CO_2$ and VD/VT were increased during exercise. No simultaneous measurements were made of distribution of ventilation. As predicted from the minute ventilation equation above, the slope of $\dot{V}E$ vs. $\dot{V}CO_2$ was increased in the group of heart failure patients in which VD/VT was increased. Lewis et al.,[19] using similar techniques, concluded that the increased ventilatory cost of CO_2 elimination found in certain patients with CHF is related to the inability to optimize the relative distribution of lung perfusion to ventilation during exercise, despite that fact the patients with the higher slopes started with better V/Q matching in their study.

Interventions that Alter $\dot{V}E$ vs. $\dot{V}CO_2$ Slope

The study of interventions that can alter the $\dot{V}E$ vs. $\dot{V}CO_2$ slope may help us understand the mechanism of the increased slope. One of the first interventions shown to be able to reduce the slope was exercise training,[20] an intervention that has been shown to improve exercise capacity and perhaps even survival.[21] How training has this effect is uncertain, but the consensus of most experts is that most of the established training effects in CHF relate to effects on peripheral muscle and blood flow.

L-arginine, the precursor to nitric oxide (NO) and hence involved in endothelial function, has been shown to reduce the slope.[22] Many have argued that L-arginine has this effect by increasing pulmonary blood flow; however, the fact that it also increases peripheral blood flow[23] does not establish that this is the predominant mode of action. Other interventions also appear able to improve the elevated $\dot{V}E$ vs. $\dot{V}CO_2$ slope. Reindl and Kleber[24] showed that modification of diuretic and angiotensin-converting enzyme inhibitor therapy over a few weeks improved the $\dot{V}E$ vs. $\dot{V}CO_2$ slope, although whether this was via a change in dead space ventilation was not established, despite the authors' belief that this was the mechanism.

In a randomized, controlled study of CHF, Matsumoto and colleagues[25] showed that inhaled NO but not isosorbide dinitrate could reduce the ventilatory response to exercise, suggesting more persuasively that pulmonary vasodilatation per se could alter the $\dot{V}E$ vs. $\dot{V}CO_2$ slope. This is also supported by a second study of inhaled NO.[26] The finding that endogenous levels of exhaled NO significantly predict exercise capacity supports the concept that NO itself may be involved in the physiological regulation of pulmonary blood flow that in part determines factors that impact on exercise capacity.[27] Whether this is via VD/VT and thereby $\dot{V}E$ vs. $\dot{V}CO_2$ slope is not certain, but it should be revealed by simultaneous arterial PCO_2 measurements.

Banning et al.[28] showed that the possibly positively inotropic vasodilator flosequinan improved exercise capacity associated with a reduction in the $\dot{V}E$ vs. $\dot{V}CO_2$ slope, a feature they also described for rate-responsive pacing in a small subset of CHF patients.[29] Reindl et al.[30] have supported an important role for deficient pulmonary vasodilator tone in the heightened $\dot{V}E$ vs. $\dot{V}CO_2$ slope by showing in 57 patients with CHF (NYHA Classes II through

IV, ejection fraction 25.6±10.4%) that the $\dot{V}E$ vs $\dot{V}CO_2$ slope correlated negatively with exercise tolerance (maximal $\dot{V}O_2$, r=-0.67) and cardiac output (r=-0.66) and positively with pulmonary hypertension (mean pulmonary artery pressure, r=0.69; pulmonary vascular resistance, r=0.60).

Predicting Prognosis in CHF

Many parameters have been proposed for predicting prognosis in CHF. These include hemodynamic, neurohormonal, electrocardiographic,[31] and treatment parameters.[32] The prognostic value of cardiopulmonary physiological parameters has also been extensively addressed. Robbins and colleagues[33] showed in 470 CHF patients followed for 1.5 years that in univariate analyses predictors of death included high $\dot{V}E$ vs. $\dot{V}CO_2$ slope, low chronotropic index, low $\dot{V}O_2$, low resting systolic blood pressure, and older age. In multivariate analyses, the only independent predictors of death were high $\dot{V}E$ vs. $\dot{V}CO_2$ slope (adjusted relative risk [RR] 3.20, 95% confidence interval [CI] 1.95 to 5.26, p<0.0001) and low chronotropic index (adjusted RR 1.94, 95% CI 1.18 to 3.19, p=0.0009). They concluded that the ventilatory and chronotropic responses to exercise are powerful and independent predictors of heart failure mortality.[33] In another study, Bol and colleagues[34] analyzed the all-cause mortality over a period of 6 years in 60 male CHF patients, assessing functional NYHA class, radionuclide left ventricular ejection fraction (29.2±10.4%), and peak values of heart rate, $\dot{V}O_2$, $\dot{V}CO_2$, $\dot{V}E$, AT, and exercise duration with an incremental workload test on the treadmill. $\dot{V}O_2$ relative to $\dot{V}E$ was based on the individual slopes of the regression of $\dot{V}O_2$ on $\dot{V}E$ during the first 6 minutes of exercise. These slopes with other exercise-related variables and factors such as etiology, medication, and NYHA class were analyzed with a Cox's regression method. A survival time analysis (Kaplan-Meier survival curve) was done to establish the influence of the slope of $\dot{V}E$ vs. $\dot{V}O_2$ and left ventricular ejection fraction (both split into above and below median values), as well as their interaction, on survival. From all investigated exercise-related variables, $\dot{V}E$ vs. $\dot{V}O_2$ slope was found to be the most powerful variable regarding prediction of all-cause mortality.

We showed in 303 consecutive patients with stable CHF with a median follow-up of 47 months (91 deaths) that the areas under the receiver operating characteristic curves for predicting mortality at 2 years were 0.77 for both peak $\dot{V}O_2$ and $\dot{V}E$ vs. $\dot{V}CO_2$ slope.[35] With peak $\dot{V}O_2$ and $\dot{V}E$ vs. $\dot{V}CO_2$ slope viewed as continuous variables in the Cox proportional hazards model, they were both highly significant prognostic indicators, both in univariate analysis and bivariate analysis (p<0.001 for $\dot{V}E$ vs. $\dot{V}CO_2$ slope, p<0.003 for peak $\dot{V}O_2$). Lower peak $\dot{V}O_2$ implies poorer prognosis across a range of values from 10 to 20 mL/kg/min, without a unique threshold. Gradations of elevation of the $\dot{V}E$ vs. $\dot{V}CO_2$ slope also carry prognostic information over a wide range

(30 to 55). The two parameters were comparable in terms of prognostic power, and contribute complementary prognostic information.

Many prognostic factors may be redundant, and whether a factor significantly predicts prognosis may depend on details of patient and selection. Left ventricular ejection fraction, for example, loses its prognostic value in favor of exercise capacity if patients are selected on the basis of having markedly impaired left ventricular ejection fraction. This suggests that noncardiac factors or the peripheral complications of heart failure begin to dominate the prognosis.[36]

Summary

An increased ventilatory response to CO_2 has been repeatedly demonstrated to relate to all-cause mortality in CHF populations. Although its precise physiological cause remains complicated and uncertain, these findings stress the valuable information that can be obtained by analysis of the cardiopulmonary exercise test responses in CHF patients.

References

1. Rubin SA, Brown HV. Ventilation and gas exchange during exercise in severe chronic heart failure. Am Rev Respir Dis 1984;129(2 Pt. 2):S63-S64.

2. Reindl I, Wernecke KD, Opitz C, et al. Impaired ventilatory efficiency in chronic heart failure: possible role of pulmonary vasoconstriction. Am Heart J 1998; 136:778-785.

3. Ponikowski P, Francis DP, Piepoli MF, et al. Enhanced ventilatory response to exercise in patients with chronic heart failure and preserved exercise tolerance: marker of abnormal cardiorespiratory reflex control and predictor of poor prognosis. Circulation 2001;103:967-972.

4. Clark AL, Poole-Wilson PA, Coats AJS. Relation between ventilation and carbon dioxide production in patients with chronic heart failure. J Am Coll Cardiol 1992; 20:1326-1332.

5. Sullivan MJ, Higginbotham MB, Cobb FR. Increased exercise ventilation in patients with chronic heart failure: intact ventilatory control despite hemodynamic and pulmonary abnormalities. Circulation 1988;77:552-559.

6. Johnson RL Jr. Gas exchange efficiency in congestive heart failure. II. Circulation 2001;103:916-918.

7. Clark AL, Volterrani M, Swan JW, Coats AJ. Ventilation-perfusion matching in chronic heart failure. Int J Cardiol 1995;48:259-270.

8. Piepoli M, Clark AL, Volterrani M, Adamopoulos S, Sleight P, Coats AJ. Contribution of muscle afferents to the hemodynamic, autonomic, and ventilatory responses to exercise in patients with chronic heart failure: effects of physical training. Circulation 1996;93:940-952.

9. Grieve DA, Clark AL, McCann GP, Hillis WS. The ergoreflex in patients with chronic stable heart failure. Int J Cardiol 1999;68:157-164.

10. Chua TP, Clark AL, Amadi AA, Coats AJS. Relation between chemosensitivity and the ventilatory response to exercise in chronic heart failure. J Am Coll Cardiol 1996;27:650-657.

11. Andreas S, Morguet AJ, Werner GS, Kreuzer H. Ventilatory response to exercise and to carbon dioxide in patients with heart failure. Eur Heart J 1996;17:750-755.

12. Chua TP, Ponikowski P, Harrington D, et al. Clinical correlates and prognostic significance of the ventilatory response to exercise in chronic heart failure. J Am Coll Cardiol 1997;29:1585-1590.

13. Jondeau G, Katz SD, Zohman L, et al. Active skeletal muscle mass and cardiopulmonary reserve. Failure to attain peak aerobic capacity during maximal bicycle exercise in patients with severe congestive heart failure. Circulation 1992; 86:1351-1356.

14. Franciosa JA, Ledy CL, Willen M, et al. Relation between hemodynamic and ventilatory responses in determining exercise capacity in severe congestive heart failure. Am J Cardiol 1984;53:127-134.

15. Wasserman K, Zhang YY, Gitt A, et al. Lung function and exercise gas exchange in chronic heart failure. Circulation 1997;96:2221-2227.

16. Juilliere Y, Grentzinger A, Houplon P, Demoulin S, Berder V, Suty-Selton C. Role of the etiology of cardiomyopathies on exercise capacity and oxygen consumption in patients with severe congestive heart failure. Int J Cardiol 2000; 73:251-255.

17. Chauhan A, Sridhar G, Clemens R, Krishnan B, Marciniuk DD, Gallagher CG. Role of respiratory function in exercise limitation in chronic heart failure. Chest 2000;118:53-60.

18. Wada O, Asanoi H, Miyagi K, et al. Importance of abnormal lung perfusion in excessive exercise ventilation in chronic heart failure. Am Heart J 1993; 125: 790-798.

19. Lewis NP, Banning AP, Cooper JP, et al. Impaired matching of perfusion and ventilation in heart failure detected by 133xenon. Basic Res Cardiol 1996;91(suppl 1):45-49.

20. Davey P, Meyer T, Coats A, et al. Ventilation in chronic heart failure: effects of physical training. Br Heart J 1992;68:473-477.

21. Piepoli MF, Capucci A. Exercise training in heart failure: effect on morbidity and mortality. Int J Cardiol 2000;73:3-6.

22. Banning AP, Prendergast B. Intravenous L-arginine reduces $\dot{V}_E/\dot{V}_{CO_2}$ slope acutely in patients with severe chronic heart failure. Eur J Heart Fail 1999; 1:187-190.

23. Kanaya Y, Nakamura M, Kobayashi N, Hiramori K. Effects of L-arginine on lower limb vasodilator reserve and exercise capacity in patients with chronic heart failure. Heart 1999;81:512-517.

24. Reindl I, Kleber FX. Exertional hyperpnea in patients with chronic heart failure is a reversible cause of exercise intolerance. Basic Res Cardiol 1996;91(suppl 1):37-43.

25. Matsumoto A, Momomura S, Sugiura S, et al. Effect of inhaled nitric oxide on gas exchange in patients with congestive heart failure. A randomized, controlled trial. Ann Intern Med 1999;130:40-44.

26. Bocchi EA, Auler JO, Guimaraes GV, et al. Nitric oxide inhalation reduces pulmonary tidal volume during exercise in severe chronic heart failure. Am Heart J 1997;134:737-744.

27. Clini E, Volterrani M, Pagani M, et al. Endogenous nitric oxide in patients with chronic heart failure (CHF): relation to functional impairment and nitrate-containing therapies. Int J Cardiol 2000;73:123-130.

28. Banning AP, Ramsey MW, Jones EA, et al. Flosequinan in chronic heart failure: how is exercise capacity improved? Eur J Clin Pharmacol 1996;51:133-138.

29. Banning AP, Lewis NP, Northridge DB, Elborn JS, Hendersen AH. Perfusion/ventilation mismatch during exercise in chronic heart failure: an investigation of circulatory determinants. Br Heart J 1995;74:27-33.

30. Reindl I, Wernecke KD, Opitz C, et al. Impaired ventilatory efficiency in chronic heart failure: possible role of pulmonary vasoconstriction. Am Heart J 1998;136:778-785.

31. Shamim W, Francis DP, Yousufuddin M, et al. Intraventricular conduction delay: a prognostic marker in chronic heart failure. Int J Cardiol 1999;70:171-178.

32. Harjai KJ, Dinshaw HK, Nunez E, et al. The prognostic implications of outpatient diuretic dose in heart failure. Int J Cardiol 1999;71:219-225.

33. Robbins M, Francis G, Pashkow FJ, et al. Ventilatory and heart rate responses to exercise: better predictors of heart failure mortality than peak oxygen consumption. Circulation 1999;100:2411-2417.

34. Bol E, de Vries WR, Mosterd WL, Wielenga RP, Coats AJ. Cardiopulmonary exercise parameters in relation to all-cause mortality in patients with chronic heart failure. Int J Cardiol 2000;72:255-263.

35. Francis DP, Shamim W, Davies LC, et al. Cardiopulmonary exercise testing for prognosis in chronic heart failure: continuous and independent prognostic value from $\dot{V}E/\dot{V}CO_2$ slope and peak $\dot{V}O_2$. Eur Heart J 2000;21:154-161.

36. Niebauer J, Clark AL, Anker SD, Coats AJ. Three year mortality in heart failure patients with very low left ventricular ejection fractions. Int J Cardiol 1999;70:245-247.

5

Peak V̇o₂, Anaerobic Threshold, and Ventilatory Equivalent as Predictors of Survival in Heart Failure

Anselm K. Gitt, MD, Caroline Bergmeier, MD, and Jochen Senges, MD

In patients with chronic heart failure (CHF), dyspnea on exertion is one of the main limiting factors of exercise capacity. Although the degree of exercise intolerance in these patients somehow reflects the severity of the disease, symptoms are only modestly related to functional capacity, and symptom scores underestimate the degree of functional impairment.[1]

Physical exercise requires the integration of the cardiovascular and ventilatory systems to support gas exchange and O_2 delivery to the working muscle. In CHF patients, gas transport, as the major role of the cardiovascular system, is impaired due to the reduction of systolic left ventricular function.[2,3] A progressive decrease in cardiopulmonary exercise capacity, measured as a decrease in maximal O_2 uptake (peak $\dot{V}O_2$) with increasing severity of heart failure, was first described by Weber et al.[4] The decrease in peak $\dot{V}O_2$ corresponded with the reduced maximum cardiac output and stroke volume during exercise. Cardiopulmonary exercise testing (CPET) with gas exchange measurement was described as an objective and safe noninvasive method for characterizing cardiac reserve and functional status in CHF patients.

In recent years, peak $\dot{V}O_2$ was found to predict survival in CHF[5-11] as well as the ventilatory response to exercise, expressed as the slope of $\dot{V}E$ versus $\dot{V}CO_2$ ($\dot{V}E$ vs. $\dot{V}CO_2$ slope).[12,13] The current recommendations for exercise testing in CHF patients consider the directly measured $\dot{V}O_2$ during

From Wasserman K (ed): *Cardiopulmonary Exercise Testing and Cardiovascular Health.* Armonk, NY: Futura Publishing Company, Inc.; © 2002.

exercise as preferable to the estimation of metabolic equivalents[14] for describing cardiopulmonary exercise capacity and predicting prognosis in CHF. CPET with gas exchange measurement provides important prognostic information for risk stratification in CHF and is recommended as part of the criteria to select patients for heart transplantation.[14,15]

Cardiopulmonary Exercise Parameters Predicting Prognosis in CHF Patients

Peak $\dot{V}O_2$: Absolute Value

Peak $\dot{V}O_2$, and its correlation to invasive hemodynamic data, was first described in 1982 by Weber et al.[4] in patients with CHF. Based on these findings, CHF patients had been objectively classified into different functional classes (Weber classes A through D) according to the $\dot{V}O_2$ reached at maximal exercise.[4] Patients with little or no impairment of aerobic capacity (peak $\dot{V}O_2$ >20 mL/kg/min) were classified as class A, patients with severe limitation of aerobic capacity (peak $\dot{V}O_2$ <10 mL/kg/min) were classified as class D. Szlachcic et al.[11] first demonstrated the prognostic value of peak $\dot{V}O_2$ in a small cohort of 27 patients with CHF. Those patients with peak $\dot{V}O_2$ <10 mL/kg/min had a 1-year mortality of 77% as compared to only 21% in patients with peak $\dot{V}O_2$ between 10 and 18 mL/kg/min. Likoff et al.[16] followed 201 patients with CHF to evaluate the prognostic value of clinical and exercise data. Beside the left ventricular ejection fraction, peak $\dot{V}O_2$ was an independent predictor of mortality. Similar results were described in large patient populations of the Veterans Administration Heart Failure Trial (VHeFT).[5] Likoff et al.[16] reported a 36% 1-year mortality in patients with peak $\dot{V}O_2$ <13 mL/kg/min.

With the increasing number of candidates for cardiac transplantation and the limited supply of donor hearts, it became increasingly important to identify patients at high risk for death. Therefore, Mancini et al.[7] prospectively examined the use of peak $\dot{V}O_2$ for risk stratification in CHF. In a cohort of 114 heart failure patients, those with peak $\dot{V}O_2$ of >14 mL/kg/min had a 1-year survival rate similar to that of patients receiving heart transplantation. This suggested that transplantation could be safely deferred in these patients. Increasing experience has confirmed the prognostic value of peak $\dot{V}O_2$, especially in the evaluation for cardiac transplantation[17] (Table 1).[9,18-21] Based on those data, the 24th Bethesda Conference for Cardiac Transplantation[15] listed a peak $\dot{V}O_2$ <10 mL/kg/min with achievement of anaerobic metabolism as an accepted indication, and a peak $\dot{V}O_2$ ≤14 mL/kg/min and major limitation of daily activities as a probable indication for heart transplantation.

_____ **Table 1** _____

Prognostic Value of Peak $\dot{V}O_2$ in CHF Patients According to the Literature: Mortality After 1, 2, and 3 Years After Evaluation

Author	Year	CHF Patients n=	Threshold Value Peak $\dot{V}O_2$	Mortality
				1-year mortality
Szlachcic et al.[11]	1985	27	<10 mL/kg/min	77%
			10-18 mL/kg/min	21%
Likoff et al.[16]	1987	201	≤13 mL/kg/min	36%
			>13 mL/kg/min	15%
Mancini et al.[7]	1991	114	≤14 mL/kg/min	30%
			>14 ml/kg/min	6%
Stevenson et al.[9]	1996	333	<10 mL/kg/min	30%
			10-16 mL/kg/min	21%
			>16 mL/kg/min	10%
Opasich et al.[44]	1998	653	<10 mL/kg/min	36%
			10-18 mL/kg/min	13%
			>18 mL/kg/min	2%
Myers et al.[36]	1998	644	≤14 mL/kg/min	13%
			>14 mL/kg/min	5%
Gitt et al.[6]	1999	54	≤14 mL/kg/min	39%
			>14 mL/kg/min	8%
Gitt et al.[37]	2001	217	≤14 mL/kg/min	22%
			>14 mL/kg/min	5%
				2-year mortality
Francis et al.[22]	2000	303	<13 mL/kg/min	48%
			13-16.5 mL/kg/min	32%
			16.6-21.6 mL/kg/min	12%
			>21.6 mL/kg/min	4%
				3-year mortality
Osada et al.[29]	1998	500	<10 mL/kg/min	25%
			10-14 mL/kg/min	32%
			>14 mL/kg/min	7%

CHF = chronic heart failure.

Table 1 shows the different outcome data of CHF patients based on different cut-off values for peak $\dot{V}O_2$. Survival decreases with impaired cardiopulmonary exercise capacity in CHF. Reduced peak $\dot{V}O_2$ implies poor prognosis across a range of values between 10 and 20 mL/kg/min.[22] Peak $\dot{V}O_2$ is a continuous predictor of mortality in CHF and does not have an absolute prognostic cut-off point for risk stratification. Nevertheless, based on the various data, peak $\dot{V}O_2$ <10 mL/kg/min identifies high-risk patients whereas peak $\dot{V}O_2$ >18 mL/kg/min identifies low-risk patients.

Peak V̇O₂: Normalized versus Absolute Value

Peak $\dot{V}O_2$ is dependent on gender as well as on age, height, and weight.[2,3,23-25] Women reach lower peak $\dot{V}O_2$ values than men. Peak $\dot{V}O_2$ decreases with age independent of gender. The absolute peak $\dot{V}O_2$ value of, for example, 14 mL/kg/min in men reflects a greater reduction in cardiopulmonary exercise capacity than the same value in women. For risk stratification based on peak $\dot{V}O_2$, these influencing parameters should be taken into account.

Peak V̇O₂ Expressed as Percent of Predicted Normal (Peak V̇O₂ %normal)

Aaronson and Mancini[26] investigated, in 272 patients with CHF who were referred for heart transplantation, whether peak $\dot{V}O_2$ %normal, rather than an absolute value, was a better predictor of survival. Normal peak $\dot{V}O_2$ was derived from standard formulas described by Wasserman et al.[3] and Astrand.[27] Neither method of determining peak $\dot{V}O_2$ %normal significantly improved the prediction of survival over peak $\dot{V}O_2$ expressed as an absolute value in the overall patient population. Only in women did peak $\dot{V}O_2$ %normal better predict survival than peak $\dot{V}O_2$ as an absolute value. Survival predictions were related equally well to peak $\dot{V}O_2$, whether expressed as %normal or as an absolute value, in men. The authors concluded that peak $\dot{V}O_2$ <14 mL/kg/min remained a reasonable guideline by which to time heart transplantation in patients with CHF.[26] In contrast to that study, Stelken et al.[19] found peak $\dot{V}O_2$ <50% of normal to be the most significant predictor of mortality in 181 heart failure patients. The 1- and 2-year survival of heart failure patients with peak $\dot{V}O_2$ <50% of normal was 74% and 43%, respectively, compared with 98% and 90% in patients with peak $\dot{V}O_2$ >50% of normal. They concluded that, in patients who achieved peak $\dot{V}O_2$ >50% of normal, heart transplantation could be safely deferred. Di Salvo et al.[28] also showed superiority of peak $\dot{V}O_2$ %normal over the nonadjusted peak $\dot{V}O_2$. Peak $\dot{V}O_2$ <30% of normal was associated with the worst prognosis, while peak $\dot{V}O_2$ >45% of normal had the best overall survival in 67 patients with advanced heart failure.

In a recent study by Osada et al.,[29] the 3-year survival rate was 93%, 77%, and 57% in heart failure patients with peak $\dot{V}O_2$ >50%, 35% to 50%, and ≤35% of normal, respectively. A multivariate analysis of female patients of this study cohort identified peak $\dot{V}O_2$ %normal, as the best predictor of survival in this subgroup. About one third of the patients (44/154) with peak $\dot{V}O_2$ <14 mL/kg/min reached peak $\dot{V}O_2$ >50% of normal; 32 of them (73%) were women. On the other hand, of the other 110 patients with peak $\dot{V}O_2$ <14 mL/kg/min and peak $\dot{V}O_2$ >50% normal, only 6% were women. Although the relative small number of events in women precluded a detailed analysis of gender differences, these data[29] confirm the findings of Aaronson and Mancini[26] that peak $\dot{V}O_2$ %normal could provide additional value for the estimation of survival in women with CHF.

Peak $\dot{V}O_2$ Adjusted for Lean Body Mass (Peak $\dot{V}O_2$ Lean)

The absolute value of peak $\dot{V}O_2$ is related to body weight. As there is a high variability in body fat content, representing metabolically inactive body mass, Osman et al.[20] examined whether the adjustment of peak $\dot{V}O_2$ to lean body mass (peak $\dot{V}O_2$ lean) could more accurately discriminate outcomes in 225 consecutive CHF patients. Peak $\dot{V}O_2$ lean ≤19 mL/kg/min was a better predictor of outcome than the unadjusted peak $\dot{V}O_2$, especially in obese patients and in women.

Ventilatory Efficiency ($\dot{V}E$ vs. $\dot{V}CO_2$ Slope)

The main exercise-limiting symptom in CHF is dyspnea. The early onset of anaerobic metabolism in heart failure patients, with additional production of CO_2, increases the ventilatory drive. In a multicenter study, Wasserman et al.[30] showed that the increase in minute ventilation ($\dot{V}E$) was predominantly caused by an increase in dead space ventilation due to high ventilation/perfusion mismatching and an increase in CO_2 output ($\dot{V}CO_2$) relative to $\dot{V}O_2$ resulting from HCO_3^- buffering of lactic acid. In 1992, Metra et al.[31] first described the increase of $\dot{V}E$ relative to $\dot{V}CO_2$ during exercise in CHF patients (Fig. 1), expressed as the $\dot{V}E$ vs. $\dot{V}CO_2$ slope, which is calculated by linear regression analysis of the breath-by-breath data, excluding the nonlinear part of the data after the onset of ventilatory compensation for metabolic acidosis. The $\dot{V}E$ vs. $\dot{V}CO_2$ slope (ventilatory efficiency) represents the degree of ventilation/perfusion mismatching and is closely related to symptomatology in patients with advanced CHF.[32,33] The ventilatory efficiency is a sensitive objective marker of the hyperventilation in heart failure patients. In a longitudinal study of heart failure patients, Kleber et al.[33] reported a decrease of the $\dot{V}E$ vs. $\dot{V}CO_2$ slope due to a decrease of dead space ventilation by drug therapy.

As the ventilatory efficiency decreases with severity of heart failure, Chua et al.[12] examined its prognostic significance in CHF. Based on data of normal controls, they chose a threshold value of $\dot{V}E$ vs. $\dot{V}CO_2$ slope >34 for identification of high-risk patients. In a multivariate analysis, the $\dot{V}E$ vs. $\dot{V}CO_2$ slope >34 gave additional prognostic information beyond peak $\dot{V}O_2$ and could discriminate patients at high risk (Fig. 2). Similar findings were reported by Kleber et al.,[13] using a threshold value of $\dot{V}E$ vs. $\dot{V}CO_2$ slope >130% of the predicted normal value[34] (Fig. 3). Pardaens et al.,[35] however,

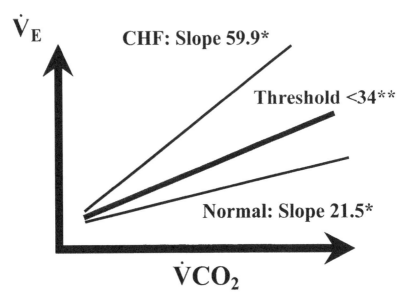

Figure 1. Increase in minute ventilation expressed as the slope of the increase of $\dot{V}_E$ relative to $\dot{V}CO_2$ in chronic heart failure patients as compared with normal subjects (*From Metra et al.[31]). Chua et al.[12] first described the prognostic significance of the ventilatory response to exercise in chronic heart failure with a threshold value of $\dot{V}_E$ vs. $\dot{V}CO_2$ slope >34 indicating impaired prognosis.

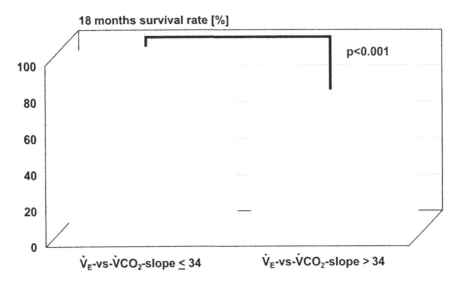

Figure 2. Eighteen-month survival rate of 173 heart failure patients as related to ventilatory efficiency, expressed as the slope of $\dot{V}_E$ vs. $\dot{V}CO_2$.[12] The threshold value used to identify high risk was a $\dot{V}_E$ vs. $\dot{V}CO_2$ slope >34.

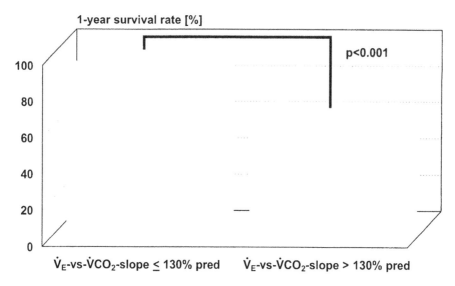

Figure 3. One-year survival rate of 142 heart failure patients dependent on the ventilatory efficiency.[13] The threshold value used to identify high risk was a V̇E vs. V̇CO₂ slope >130% of predicted normal value.

failed to demonstrate any significant advantage in risk stratification of CHF patients from the V̇E vs. V̇CO₂ slope over peak V̇O₂.

In contrast to peak V̇O₂, the ventilatory efficiency can be achieved by submaximal exercise. The ventilatory efficiency therefore cannot be influenced by premature termination of exercise. If peak V̇O₂ is reached, the ventilatory efficiency provides additional prognostic information beyond that provided by peak V̇O₂.

Anaerobic Threshold (V̇O₂ *AT*)

Peak V̇O₂ might be underestimated because of reduced patient motivation as well as by premature termination of exercise by the examiner. The anaerobic threshold, determined by gas exchange (V̇O₂ *AT*), measures the sustainable V̇O₂ of the patient and is an objective parameter of cardiopulmonary exercise capacity that can be derived from a submaximal exercise test. It therefore is independent of the above influences.[3] The existing studies concentrated on peak V̇O₂ for risk stratification of CHF patients. Kleber et al.[13] briefly reported that V̇O₂ *AT* <10 mL/kg/min could discriminate patients at high risk in a population of 142 heart failure patients. This analysis concentrated only on the prognostic value of the V̇E vs. V̇CO₂ slope and peak V̇O₂. It did not further describe the use of V̇O₂ *AT* in comparison or combination with other prognostic parameters. Myers et al.[36] followed 644 heart failure patients over 10 years after cardiopulmonary exercise evaluation. The nonsurvivors reached lower V̇O₂ *AT* values than the survivors (11.5±3.9 vs.

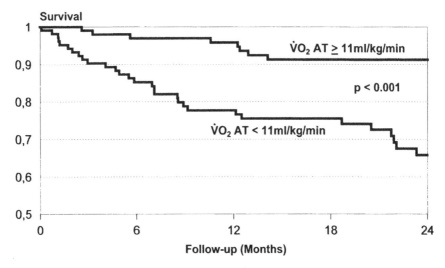

Figure 4. Kaplan-Meier survival curves using $\dot{V}O_2$ AT <11 mL/min/kg as cut-off value for the identification of increased risk of death.[37]

10.7±3.8, p=0.02). Among the exercise parameters, $\dot{V}O_2$ AT was a significant predictor of death in CHF beside peak $\dot{V}O_2$ and peak watts.[36] The authors concluded that $\dot{V}O_2$ AT might play a role in patients with heart failure who may not be able to perform symptom-limited maximal exercise test. In such patients, a submaximal exercise test could determine $\dot{V}O_2$ AT instead of peak $\dot{V}O_2$ for risk stratification; however, a cut-off to identify heart failure patients who are at a similar risk to that in peak $\dot{V}O_2$ does not exist.

In a prospective study of 217 consecutive heart failure patients, we determined the predictive value of $\dot{V}O_2$ AT <11 mL/kg/min, the ventilatory efficiency $\dot{V}E$ vs. $\dot{V}CO_2$ slope >34, and the combination of $\dot{V}O_2$ AT and the ventilatory efficiency for estimating the short-term (6 months) and long-term (2-year) survival (A.K. Gitt et al. unpublished data, 2001). Focusing on the first 6 months of follow-up after the initial evaluation, the best single predictor of early mortality (6 months) was $\dot{V}O_2$ AT <11 mL/kg/min with a 5.3-fold increased risk of death within 6 months. Patients with peak $\dot{V}O_2$ ≤14 mL/kg/min had a 3-fold increased risk, and patients with $\dot{V}E$ vs. $\dot{V}CO_2$ slope >34 had a 4.8-fold increased risk of early death. $\dot{V}O_2$ AT <11 mL/kg/min discriminated patients at increased risk of death during the entire follow-up of median 644 days (Fig. 4).

Combination of Submaximal Exercise Parameters: $\dot{V}O_2$ AT and $\dot{V}E$ vs. $\dot{V}CO_2$ Slope

For the cohort of 217 consecutive heart failure patients (A.K. Gitt et al. unpublished data, 2001), the diagnostic test analysis for the different single and combined cardiopulmonary predictors of 6-month mortality showed

_____ Table 2 _____

Diagnostic Test Analysis: Prediction of Death within 6 Months/Within Total Follow-Up

CPX Parameter	Sensitivity (%)	Specificity (%)	NPV (%)	PPV (%)
Peak V̇O₂ ≤14 mL/kg/min	70/65	59/72	95/89	14/37
Peak V̇O₂ ≤50% normal	35/77	73/46	92/83	11/37
V̇O₂ AT <11 mL/kg/min	83/56	52/78	97/90	14/33
V̇E vs. V̇CO₂ slope >34	75/65	62/64	96/86	16/34
Peak V̇O₂ ≤14 + V̇E vs. V̇CO₂ slope >34	77/71	65/75	96/90	21/44
V̇O₂ AT <11 + V̇E vs. V̇CO₂ slope >34	86/68	62/81	97/92	20/42

AT = anaerobic threshold; CPX = cardiopulmonary exercise; NPV = negative predictive value; PPV = positive predictive value.

that the combination of V̇E vs. V̇CO₂ slope >34 and V̇O₂ AT <11 mL/kg/min was superior to the single cardiopulmonary parameter with positive predictive values of 20 and 42 in predicting mortality within 6 months and within the entire follow-up of median 644 days, respectively (Table 2, Fig. 5). Mortality during the entire follow-up was highest in patients with simultaneously impaired exercise capacity and ventilatory efficiency (Table 3). With special respect to mortality within 6 months after the initial evaluation and after correction for other risk factors such as gender, age, left ventricular function, and New York Heart Association functional class, the combination of V̇E vs. V̇CO₂ slope >34 with V̇O₂ AT <11 mL/kg/min identified patients with a 6.5-fold increased risk.

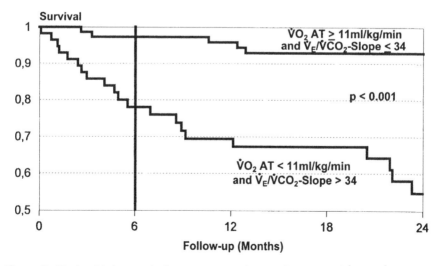

Figure 5. Kaplan-Meier survival curves using the combination of V̇E vs. V̇CO₂ slope >34 and V̇O₂ AT <11 mL/kg/min as cut-off-values for the identification of increased risk of death (A.K. Gitt et al. unpublished data, 2001).

_____ Table 3 _____

Mortality Within 6 Months and "Long Term" as Related to Selected Threshold Values for Grading Exercise Impairment

Threshold Value	6-Month Mortality	Long-Term Mortality (median 644 days)
Peak $\dot{V}O_2$ ≤14 mL/kg/min	14.4%	37.1%
Peak $\dot{V}O_2$ ≤50% normal	11.3%	37.1%
$\dot{V}O_2$ AT <11 mL/kg/min	14.2%	33.0%
$\dot{V}E$ vs. $\dot{V}CO_2$ slope >34	16.1%	34.4%
Peak $\dot{V}O_2$ ≤14 + $\dot{V}E$ vs. $\dot{V}CO_2$ slope >34	21.3%	44.3%
$\dot{V}O_2$ AT <11 + $\dot{V}E$ vs. $\dot{V}CO_2$ slope >34	20.3%	42.4%

CPET for Risk Stratification of Heart Failure Patients in the Era of Beta-Adrenergic Blockade

Large randomized trials with beta-adrenergic blocker therapy in CHF patients demonstrated a significant improvement in symptomatology as well as in outcome.[37-41] Beta-adrenergic blockade reduces $\dot{V}O_2$ at the anaerobic threshold and at peak exercise. Beta-adrenergic blocker treatment will improve outcome and will reduce peak $\dot{V}O_2$ at the same time. In patients with CHF, beta-adrenergic blockade therefore might interfere with the concept of risk stratification by CPET. Most of the existing data on prognostic evaluation of heart failure by gas exchange measurements were collected when beta-adrenergic blockade had even been contraindicated in CHF.[7,13,16,29] In recently published studies, the reported use of beta-adrenergic blockers in heart failure patients, evaluated by CPET, was low with only 12%,[21] 16%,[35] and 31%.[20] Other investigators[35] did not give information on treatment of their study population despite the known beneficial effects of angiotensin-converting enzyme inhibitors and beta-adrenergic blockers on outcome of CHF.

In our study population of 217 consecutive patients with CHF, evaluated by CPET, 95 patients (43%) were receiving chronic beta-adrenergic blocker therapy.[42] We examined the prognostic value of peak $\dot{V}O_2$, $\dot{V}O_2$ AT, and the ventilatory efficiency in patients with and without beta-adrenergic blocker treatment. The ability of peak $\dot{V}O_2$, $\dot{V}O_2$ AT, and the $\dot{V}E$ vs. $\dot{V}CO_2$ slope to predict mortality at 24 months was better without than with chronic beta-blocker treatment in CHF patients (Fig. 6). All parameters could predict impaired outcome in patients without beta-adrenergic blocker therapy but failed to predict impaired prognosis in patients with beta-blocker therapy (Fig. 7).

Although our data were not obtained from a randomized trial, they raise the question of whether the established threshold values are still applicable for risk stratification of CHF patients in the era of beta-adrenergic

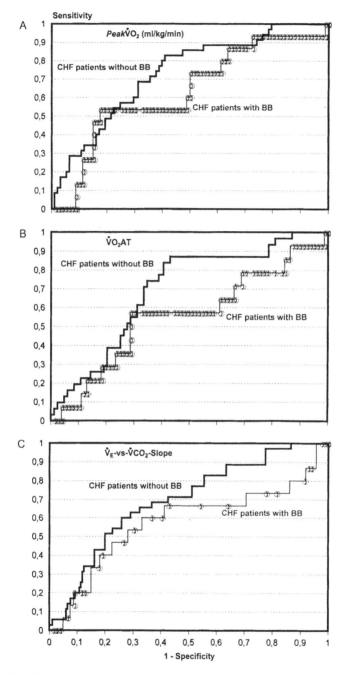

Figure 6. Receiver operating characteristic curves showing the relationship between sensitivity relative to the specificity for the ability of peak $\dot{V}o_2$ (**A**), $\dot{V}o_2$ *AT* (**B**), and $\dot{V}_E$ vs. $\dot{V}co_2$ slope (**C**) to predict mortality at 24 months in chronic heart failure patients with and without chronic beta-adrenergic blocker treatment. As sensitivity increases past 50%, specificity is lost in the blockaded patients.

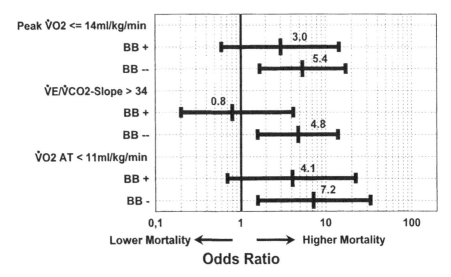

Figure 7. Cardiopulmonary predictors of mortality within 24 months in patients with chronic heart failure without (BB--) and with (BB+) chronic beta-adrenergic blocker treatment: univariate analysis. Numbers are odds ratios. Bars are 95% CI.

blockade therapy. Risk stratification in CHF by use of CPET must be reevaluated in patients with "modern" medical treatment, including beta-adrenergic blockers.

Summary

Despite recent advances in pharmacological treatment of patients with CHF, mortality in patients with severe heart failure remains high. Reliable risk stratification therefore is a continuing challenge as the number of candidates for cardiac transplantation in end-stage disease is increasing and the supply of donor hearts is limited.

Peak $\dot{V}O_2$ has been widely introduced in the risk stratification of patients with CHF. For the past 10 years, the cut-off value for the identification of patients at risk has been peak $\dot{V}O_2$ <14 mL/kg/min. Adjustment of peak $\dot{V}O_2$ (%normal) only provided advantages in women and in obese patients.

In contrast to peak $\dot{V}O_2$, the anaerobic threshold ($\dot{V}O_2$ AT), a measure of sustainable aerobic capacity, and the ventilatory efficiency ($\dot{V}E$ vs. $\dot{V}CO_2$ slope below the ventilatory compensation point) can be determined from submaximal exercise testing and cannot be influenced by the motivation of the patient. Both parameters were found to predict survival in CHF patients as well as peak $\dot{V}O_2$. With its simultaneous measurement, CPET provides two independent and reliable parameters for risk stratification in CHF. The combination of $\dot{V}O_2$ AT and $\dot{V}E$ vs. $\dot{V}CO_2$ slope was found to best predict 6-month mortality and therefore might be used in identifying patients at high risk of early death who should be listed for early cardiac transplantation.

References

1. Wilson JR, Hanamanthu S, Chomsky DB, Davis SF. Relationship between exertional symptoms and functional capacity in patients with heart failure. J Am Coll Cardiol 1999;33:1943-1947.

2. Wasserman K, Whipp BJ. Exercise physiology in health and disease. Am Rev Respir Dis 1975;112:219-249.

3. Wasserman K, Hansen JE, Sue DY, Whipp BJ, Casaburi R. Principles of Exercise Testing and Interpretation. 2nd ed. Malvern, PA: Lea & Febiger; 1994.

4. Weber KT, Kinasewitz GT, Janicki JS, Fishman AP. Oxygen utilization and ventilation during exercise in patients with chronic cardiac failure. Circulation 1982; 65:1213-1223.

5. Cohn JN, Johnson GR, Shabetai R, et al. Ejection fraction, peak exercise oxygen consumption, cardiothoracic ratio, ventricular arrhythmias, and plasma norepinephrine as determinants of prognosis in heart failure. The V-HeFT VA Cooperative Studies Group. Circulation 1993;87(6 suppl):VI5-VI16.

6. Gitt AK, Bergmeier C, Winkler R, et al. Prognostische Bedeutung der maximalen O₂-Aufnahme bei chronischer Herzinsuffizienz. Atemw-Lungenkrkh 1999; 25: 497-502.

7. Mancini DM, Eisen H, Kussmaul W, Mull R, Edmunds LHJ, Wilson JR. Value of peak exercise oxygen consumption for optimal timing of cardiac transplantation in ambulatory patients with heart failure. Circulation 1991;83:778-786.

8. Mancini DM. Cardiopulmonary exercise testing for heart transplant candidate selection. Cardiologia 1997;42:579-584.

9. Stevenson LW. Role of exercise testing in the evaluation of candidates for cardiac transplantation. In: Wasserman K (ed): Exercise Gas Exchange in Heart Disease. Armonk, New York: Futura Publishing Co.; 1996:271-286.

10. Stevenson LW. Selection and management of candidates for heart transplantation. Curr Opin Cardiol 1996;11:166-173.

11. Szlachcic J, Massie BM, Kramer BL, Topic N, Tubau J. Correlates and prognostic implication of exercise capacity in chronic congestive heart failure. Am J Cardiol 1985;55:1037-1042.

12. Chua TP, Ponikowski P, Harrington D, et al. Clinical correlates and prognostic significance of the ventilatory response to exercise in chronic heart failure. J Am Coll Cardiol 1997;29:1585-1590.

13. Kleber FX, Vietzke G, Wernecke KD, et al. Impairment of ventilatory efficiency in heart failure: prognostic impact. Circulation 2000;101:2803-2809.

14. Working Group on Cardiac Rehabilitation & Exercise Physiology and Working Group on Heart Failure of the European Society of Cardiology. Recommendations for exercise testing in chronic heart failure patients. Eur Heart J 2001;22:37-45.

15. Mudge GH, Goldstein S, Addonizio LJ, et al. 24th Bethesda Conference: cardiac transplantation. Task Force 3: recipient guidelines/prioritization. J Am Coll Cardiol 1993;22:21-31.

16. Likoff MJ, Chandler SL, Kay HR. Clinical determinants of mortality in chronic congestive heart failure secondary to idiopathic dilated or to ischemic cardiomyopathy. Am J Cardiol 1987;59:634-638.

17. Stevenson LW. Advanced congestive heart failure. Inpatient treatment and selection for cardiac transplantation. Postgrad Med 1993;94:97-100, 103-107, 112.

18. Stevenson LW, Steimle AE, Fonarow G, et al. Improvement in exercise capacity of candidates awaiting heart transplantation. J Am Coll Cardiol 1995;25:163-170.

19. Stelken AM, Younis LT, Jennison SH, et al. Prognostic value of cardiopulmonary exercise testing using percent achieved of predicted peak oxygen uptake for patients with ischemic and dilated cardiomyopathy. J Am Coll Cardiol 1996; 27:345-352.

20. Osman AF, Mehra MR, Lavie CJ, Nunez E, Milani RV. The incremental prognostic importance of body fat adjusted peak oxygen consumption in chronic heart failure. J Am Coll Cardiol 2000;36:2126-2131.

21. Myers J, Gullestad L, Vagelos R, et al. Clinical, hemodynamic, and cardiopulmonary exercise test determinants of survival in patients referred for evaluation of heart failure. Ann Intern Med 1998;129:286-293.

22. Francis DP, Shamim W, Davies LC, et al. Cardiopulmonary exercise testing for prognosis in chronic heart failure: continuous and independent prognostic value from V_E/V_{CO_2} slope and peak V_{O_2}. Eur Heart J 2000;21:154-161.

23. Astrand I, Astrand PO, Hallback I, Kilbom A. Reduction in maximal oxygen uptake with age. J Appl Physiol 1973;35:649-654.

24. Astrand PO. Human physical fitness with special reference to sex and age. Am Physiol Soc 1956;36:307.

25. Hansen JE, Sue DY, Wasserman K. Predicted values for clinical exercise testing. Am Rev Respir Dis 1984;129(2 Pt. 2):S49-S55.

26. Aaronson KD, Mancini DM. Is percentage of predicted maximal exercise oxygen consumption a better predictor of survival than peak exercise oxygen consumption for patients with severe heart failure? J Heart Lung Transplant 1995; 14: 981-989.

27. Astrand PO. Quantification of exercise capability and evaluation of physical capacity in man. Prog Cardiovasc Dis 1976;19:51-67.

28. Di Salvo TG, Mathier M, Semigran MJ, Dec GW. Preserved right ventricular ejection fraction predicts exercise capacity and survival in advanced heart failure. J Am Coll Cardiol 1995;25:1143-1153.

29. Osada N, Chaitman BR, Miller LW, et al. Cardiopulmonary exercise testing identifies low risk patients with heart failure and severely impaired exercise capacity considered for heart transplantation. J Am Coll Cardiol 1998;31:577-582.

30. Wasserman K, Zhang YY, Gitt A, et al. Lung function and exercise gas exchange in chronic heart failure. Circulation 1997;96:2221-2227.

31. Metra M, Dei CL, Panina G, Visioli O. Exercise hyperventilation chronic congestive heart failure, and its relation to functional capacity and hemodynamics [see comments]. Am J Cardiol 1992;70:622-628.

32. Reindl I, Kleber FX. Exertional hyperpnea in patients with chronic heart failure is a reversible cause of exercise intolerance. Basic Res Cardiol 1996;91(suppl 1):37-43.

33. Kleber FX, Reindl I, Wernecke KD, Baumann G. Dyspnea in heart failure. In: Wasserman K (ed): Exercise Gas Exchange in Heart Disease. Armonk, New York: Futura Publishing Co., 1996:95-108.

34. Habedank D, Reindl I, Vietzke G, et al. Ventilatory efficiency and exercise tolerance in 101 healthy volunteers. Eur J Appl Physiol 1988;77:421-426.

35. Pardaens K, Van Cleemput J, Vanhaecke J, Fagard R. Peak oxygen uptake better predicts outcome than submaximal respiratory data in heart transplant candidates. Circulation 2000;101:1152-1157.

36. Myers J, Gullestad L, Vagelos R, et al. Clinical, hemodynamic, and cardiopulmonary exercise test determinants of survival in patients referred for evaluation of heart failure. Ann Intern Med 1998;129:286-293.

37. Pamboukian SV, Aminbakhsh A, Thompson CR, et al. Carvedilol improves functional class in patients with severe left ventricular dysfunction referred for heart transplantation. Clin Transplant 1999;13:426-431.

38. Packer M. Effects of beta-adrenergic blockade on survival of patients with chronic heart failure. Am J Cardiol 1997;80:46L-54L.

39. Packer M. Beta-blockade in heart failure. Basic concepts and clinical results. Am J Hypertens 1998;11:23S-37S.

40. Packer M. Do beta-blockers prolong survival in chronic heart failure? A review of the experimental and clinical evidence. Eur Heart J 1998;19(suppl B):B40-B46.

41. Cohn JN, Fowler MB, Bristow MR, et al. Safety and efficacy of carvedilol in severe heart failure. The U.S. Carvedilol Heart Failure Study Group. J Card Fail 1997;3:173-179.

42. Gitt AK, Bergmeier C, Kleemann T, et al. Different prognostic value of the oxygen-uptake and the ventilatory efficacy in the risk stratification of heart failure patients with and without chronic beta-blocker therapy. J Am Coll Cardiol. 2001;37:212A. Abstract

43. Opasich C, Pinna GD, Bobbio M, et al. Peak exercise oxygen consumption in chronic heart failure: toward efficient use in the individual patient. J Am Coll Cardiol 1998;31:766-775.

6

Abnormalities in Exercise-Derived Gas Exchange Variables Other than Peak $\dot{V}O_2$ and Anaerobic Threshold in Chronic Heart Failure

Alain Cohen-Solal, MD, PhD, Maria Tokmakova, MD, Pierre Vladimir Ennezat, MD, and Jean-Yves Tabet, MD

In the last 15 years, cardiopulmonary exercise testing has become a major tool to assess functional capacity, analyze the pathophysiology of the circulatory and ventilatory responses to exercise, assess the effects of treatments, and evaluate prognosis in patients with chronic heart failure (CHF). Peak O_2 uptake (peak $\dot{V}O_2$) and the anaerobic threshold (*AT*) are the only parameters generally looked for by cardiologists when they read the report of a test; however, many other variables, the value of which is overlooked, can be used to assess functional capacity during a test. In this chapter we review these variables.

The *slope of the $\dot{V}O_2$/time or $\dot{V}O_2$/work rate response* during exercise has appeared as an index of circulatory response during exercise.[1-4] It reflects the oxygen cost of carrying out work—the more reduced the slope, the more the anaerobic metabolism and severity of the circulatory failure (Table 1, Fig. 1). This is due to the fact that at each work rate, the time to reach a steady state is longer in CHF patients than in normal subjects. When stages of 4 or 5 minutes in duration are used, $\dot{V}O_2$ at each stage is generally identical in patients and in normal subjects. In normal subjects, the $\dot{V}O_2$/work rate relationship is approximately 10 mL/min/W. In CHF patients, it can decrease to <8 mL/min/W. This index is best applied with ramp protocols on

From Wasserman K (ed): *Cardiopulmonary Exercise Testing and Cardiovascular Health.* Armonk, NY: Futura Publishing Company, Inc.; © 2002.

_____ Table 1 _____

Oxygen Consumption* at Increasing Work Rate†, and ΔV̇o₂/ΔW as Related to Grade of Severity of CHF

Grade of CHF	Rest	20W	40W	60W	80W	100W	120W	ΔV̇o₂/ΔW (mL/min/W)
Controls	4.1	9.0	11.4	14.1	17.0	19.8	22.7	11.1 ± 0.4
CHF-A	4.3	9.0	11.2	14.0	17.2	19.3	21.7	11.4 ± 1.5
CHF-B	4.3	8.3	10.4	12.9	15.0‡	16.7‡	18.2‡	10.2 ± 1.6
CHF-CD	3.9	7.4‡	9.3‡	10.8‡	12.2‡	13.8‡	14.2‡	8.8 ± 2.1‡
CHF avg.	4.2	8.3	10.4‡	12.9‡	15.5‡	18.1‡	20.7‡	10.2 ± 2.0‡

*mL/kg/min; †Watts (W).
ΔV̇o₂/ΔW = increase in V̇o₂ per increase in W; CHF = chronic heart failure.
A is least severe and D is most severe (Weber's classification).
‡p<0.05 versus controls. From reference 3.

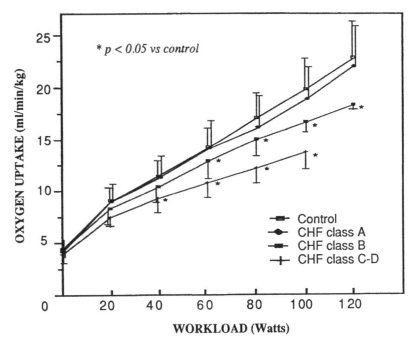

Figure 1. Slope of the relationship between O_2 uptake and workload during exercise in normal subjects and in patients with chronic heart failure (CHF). Adapted from reference 3.

bicycle, and calculated only after some minutes of zero-workload pedaling. Its main value is that it can be determined even if exercise is submaximal.

The *oxygen pulse* reflects the capacity of the heart to deliver O_2 per beat. It is calculated from the V̇o₂ divided by heart rate and is equal to the product of stroke volume and the arterial-mixed venous O_2 difference, $C(a-v)O_2$. Peak oxygen pulse is generally low in CHF during exercise because stroke volume is reduced and $C(a-v)O_2$ cannot widen enough to compensate for the reduced exercise cardiac output at peak exercise. The O_2 pulse response profile also is abnormal in CHF. As $C(a-v)O_2$ always increases during exercise, a plateau of O_2 pulse presumably reflects a decrease in stroke volume as $C(a-v)O_2$ increases, or the reaching of a maximum $C(a-v)O_2$ during early exercise. In fact, the increase in O_2 pulse is more dependent on $C(a-v)O_2$ difference than on stroke volume during exercise because stroke volume only increases by 50% in normal subjects and may not increase at all in patients with CHF in response to exercise. In contrast, $C(a-v)O_2$ can increase as much as 300% in normal subjects, but usually less in patients because of a high resting $C(a-v)O_2$. While the peak $\dot{V}O_2$ has been found to have prognostic value, we have found the O_2 pulse at peak exercise not to have prognostic value in CHF patients.[5]

The *kinetics of recovery in* $\dot{V}O_2$ has also emerged in the recent years as an interesting variable.[6] In normal subjects, $\dot{V}O_2$ rapidly declines after exercise.[7] The kinetics of this recovery has been found to correlate with the recovery of energy stores in the active muscles.[8] Thus, it describes the rate of recovery of phosphocreatine (PCr) levels after exercise as well as the recovery of the blood and the tissue O_2 stores. The kinetics of recovery of $\dot{V}O_2$ does not appear to be affected by workload in normal subjects.[9,10] As it has been reported that the recovery of energy stores in skeletal muscles is prolonged after exercise in CHF,[11] it was tempting to hypothesize that repayment of the so-called "oxygen debt"[12] is prolonged in patients, in parallel with the delayed recovery of energy stores in peripheral muscles.

In normal subjects, the kinetics of recovery of $\dot{V}O_2$ is generally considered to fit a single exponential curve[13-16] but, in most cases, a multiexponential fitting seems more suitable.[16,17] When plotting $\dot{V}O_2$ versus time during the first 3 minutes of recovery as a single exponential (a multiexponential fitting is more accurate after 3 minutes even in normal subjects[16]), one can assess the slope of the single exponential regression, the slope k of the exponential relationship being derived by the equation:

$$\dot{V}O_2 (\tau) = A.e^{-kt} + C$$

where k, the rate constant, is the slope of the curve, A a parameter, and C the asymptotic baseline value. Tau, the time constant, defined as $1/k$ and $T\frac{1}{2}_{(exp)} = 0.693$ Tau are used to characterize the kinetics. A simpler way of characterizing recovery kinetics is by simply measuring the half-time of recovery, $T\frac{1}{2}$, i.e., the time required for a 50% fall in the peak value. This method has the advantage of being independent of the regression model chosen (Figs. 2 and 3). $T\frac{1}{2}_{(exp)}$ $\dot{V}O_2$ and $T\frac{1}{2}$ $\dot{V}O_2$ are closely correlated (r= 0.86, p<0.0001) in our experience.[6]

The kinetics of $\dot{V}O_2$ recovery is also largely independent of the motivation of the patient. $T\frac{1}{2}$ $\dot{V}O_2$ in *normal subjects* after 100%, 75%, and 50% of peak exercise tests were measured at 57±6, 57±6, and 53±8 seconds,

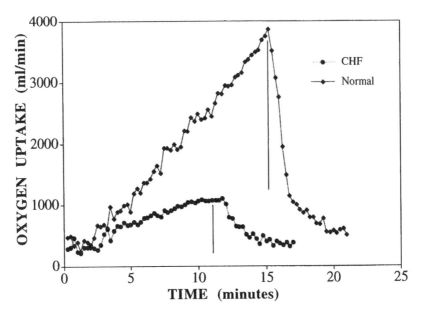

Figure 2. $\dot{V}O_2$ recovery profiles in a chronic heart failure (CHF) patient and a normal subject after performing a progressively increasing work rate exercise test.

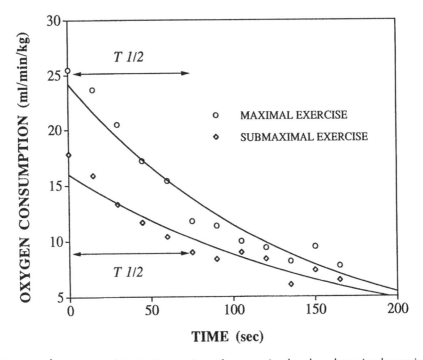

Figure 3. $\dot{V}O_2$ recovery kinetics in a patient after a maximal and a submaximal exercise. Despite the fact that peak $\dot{V}O_2$ differs (16 vs. 24 mL/kg/min), the half-times of $\dot{V}O_2$ recovery are roughly the same. From reference 6.

respectively. Coefficients of variation between 100% and 75% and between 100% and 50% of peak workload levels were 5.7% and 8.6%, respectively. When *CHF patients* were considered, the kinetics of recovery did not change significantly when they exercised at 100% or 75% of peak workload. $T^{1/2}$ $\dot{V}O_2$ were 93 ± 20 and 93 ± 20 seconds, respectively. The coefficient of variation of $T^{1/2}$ $\dot{V}O_2$ was 13.8%. There was, however, a significant difference in $T^{1/2}$ $\dot{V}O_2$ between 100% and 50% of peak workload: 103 ± 23 and 93 ± 19 seconds, respectively (p=0.02) (coefficient of variation 14%).[6] These characteristics may be of great value when assessing patients, who often stop exercising before their maximum workload because of symptoms or poor motivation. Thus, the kinetics of recovery of O_2 consumption is probably similar to PCr recovery and can be determined with confidence even for a submaximal exercise test.

There is a negative relationship between $T^{1/2}$ $\dot{V}O_2$ and peak $\dot{V}O_2$ (r=-0.65, p<0.0001).[6] A $T^{1/2}$ $\dot{V}O_2$ >100 seconds (2 standard deviations above the mean value of the control group) appears to be associated with abnormal O_2 transport and/or utilization (Fig. 4), even in case of submaximal exercise.

Various factors may account for the increase in $T^{1/2}$ $\dot{V}O_2$ in CHF, and slowed replenishment of energy stores in peripheral muscles may be the most important. The half-time of recovery of PCr, or of Pi/PCr after exercise, was found to be increased in patients with CHF[18-20] and, conversely, decreased in athletes.[21] In our study, $T^{1/2}$ $\dot{V}O_2$ correlated with $T^{1/2}$ Pi/PCr (measured by nuclear magnetic resonance spectroscopy during an exercise

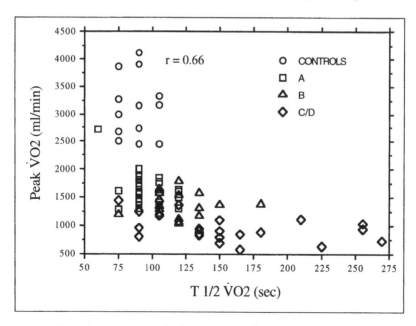

Figure 4. Relationship between $T^{1/2}$ $\dot{V}O_2$ and peak $\dot{V}O_2$ in patients with chronic heart failure; A, B, and C-D refer to Weber's functional classes. From reference 6.

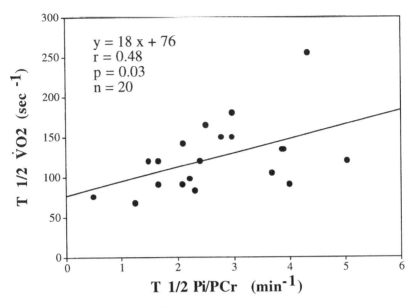

Figure 5. Relationship between $T^{1/2}$ $\dot{V}O_2$ and $T^{1/2}$ Pi/PCr (the half-time of phosphocreatine recovery within the muscle after exercise) in patients with chronic heart failure. From reference 6.

performed with one leg; r=0.62, p=0.001) (Fig. 5),[6] suggesting that the slower kinetics of replenishment of energy stores in peripheral skeletal muscles after exercise may partly account for the increase in $T^{1/2}$ $\dot{V}O_2$. The decrease in blood velocity resulting in an increased transit time between peripheral muscles and the mouth may also explain the prolongation of $\dot{V}O_2$ recovery kinetics. It is likely that during the first minutes after cessation of exercise, there is a delay between O_2 consumption measured at the peripheral muscles and the mouth that increases as heart failure worsens.[22,23] Thus, inadequate cardiac output during exercise probably accounts for the prolongation of $T^{1/2}$ $\dot{V}O_2$.[24]

Prolonged kinetics of recovery of O_2 consumption is not, however, specific to CHF. O_2 consumption recovery is shortened by training[25-27] and prolonged by bed-rest-induced deconditioning,[28] beta-adrenergic blockade,[29] and in chronic obstructive pulmonary disease.[30] Therefore, $T^{1/2}$ $\dot{V}O_2$ appears to be increased whenever transport and/or utilization of O_2 to the working muscles is impaired, such as in anemia, hypoxia, peripheral artery disease, peripheral myopathies, or simply deconditioning.

Whether this parameter is more dependent on cardiac or peripheral factors remains under debate. Recent studies have shown that in patients with mitral stenosis undergoing exercise training after percutaneous valvuloplasty, but not those who had undergone valvuloplasty alone, $T^{1/2}$ $\dot{V}O_2$ is decreased.[31] Finally, $T^{1/2}$ $\dot{V}O_2$ has also been found to have prognostic value. de Groote et al.[32] found that the kinetics of recovery of $\dot{V}O_2$ was an independent

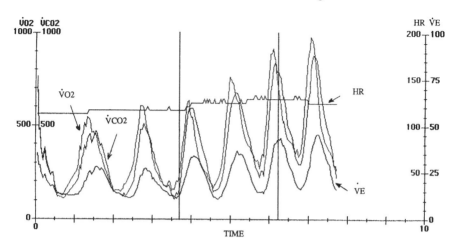

Figure 6. Example of an oscillatory pattern of ventilation, $\dot{V}O_2$ and $\dot{V}CO_2$ at rest and during the first minutes of exercise in a patient with chronic heart failure.

predictor of outcome in patients with moderately reduced peak $\dot{V}O_2$. We recently extended these observations by showing that $T^1/_2$ $\dot{V}O_2$ had a highly powerful prognostic value even in patients with severe heart failure.[33]

The *blood pressure* response is also important to consider. Osada et al.[34] showed in a large cohort of patients with CHF that the only predictors of outcome by multivariate analysis were peak $\dot{V}O_2$ (indexed by predicted values) and the blood pressure response.[35-37] This is consistent with the observation that combining the blood pressure and the cardiac output or stroke volume response has important prognostic value. In studies using invasive hemodynamic measurements during exercise, peak cardiac stroke work (the product of mean arterial pressure and stroke volume) has emerged as the most powerful predictor of outcome in these groups of patients[35-37]; however, one may question the safety as well as the necessity of performing such invasive measurements, routinely, since the impaired exercise performance is revealed by noninvasive gas exchange measurements. We recently found that the product of peak $\dot{V}O_2$ and peak systolic arterial pressure ("the circulatory power") probably has the same prognostic impact as peak cardiac output times peak arterial pressure (peak cardiac power). Peak exercise circulatory stroke work, a surrogate of peak stroke work, has less prognostic value.[33]

The presence of a poor *heart rate response*,[38] a *rebound of $\dot{V}O_2$* at the beginning of recovery,[39] or an *oscillatory ventilatory and gas exchange pattern* (Fig. 6)[40-42] is generally associated with severe functional impairment and poor prognosis. Periodic breathing is an intriguing finding in patients with severe heart failure,[40-42] and its origin remains unclear. It is attributed to primary cardiac factors by some investigators[43,44] and to primary ventilatory control factors by others.[45-48] It may persist during exercise but generally tends to disappear as work rate increases and reappear in recovery. Various studies suggested that an oscillatory pattern in ventilation was indicative of poor prognosis.[49]

Summary

When assessing the exercise response of patients with CHF, one should consider many other variables besides peak $\dot{V}O_2$ and the *AT*. The global analysis of all these parameters gives an enormous amount of information from a single test, implying that cardiopulmonary exercise testing is mandatory for the optimal evaluation of patients with CHF.

References

1. Itoh H, Taniguchi K, Koike A, Doi M. Evaluation of the severity of heart failure using ventilatory gas analysis. Circulation 1990;81(suppl II):II-31-II-37.
2. Hansen J, Sue D, Oren A, Wasserman K. Relation of oxygen uptake to work rate in normal men and men with circulatory disorders. Am J Cardiol 1987;59:669-674.
3. Cohen-Solal A, Chabernaud J, Gourgon R. Comparison of oxygen uptake during bicycle exercise in patients with chronic heart failure and in normal subjects. J Am Coll Cardiol 1990;16:80-85.
4. Myers J, Buchanan N, Walsh D, et al. A comparison of the ramp versus standard exercise protocols. J Am Coll Cardiol 1991;17:339-343.
5. Cohen-Solal A, Barnier P, Pessione F, et al. Comparison of the long term prognostic value of peak exercise oxygen uptake and peak oxygen pulse in patients with chronic heart failure. Heart 1998;78:572-576.
6. Cohen-Solal A, Laperche T, Morvan D, Geneves M, Caviezel B, Gourgon R. Prolonged kinetics of recovery of oxygen consumption and ventilatory variables after maximal graded exercise in patients with chronic heart failure. Analysis with gas exchange and NMR spectroscopy study. Circulation 1995;91:2924-2932.
7. Margaria R, Edwards H, Dill D. The possible mechanisms of contracting and paying the oxygen debt and the role of lactic acid in muscular contraction. Am J Physiol 1933;106:689-715.
8. Harris R, Edwards R, Hultman E, Nordesjo L, Nylind B, Sahlin K. The time course of phosphoryl-creatine resynthesis during recovery of the quadriceps muscle in man. Pfluegers Arch 1976;367:137-142.
9. Sapega A, Sokolow D, Graham T, Chance B. Phosphorus nuclear magnetic resonance: a non-invasive technique for the study of muscle bioenergetics during exercise. Med Sci Sports Exerc 1987;19:410-420.
10. McCully K, Strear C, Prammer M, Leigh J Jr. Recovery of PCr after exercise as an index of oxidative capacity in man. FASEB J 1990;4:A1212.
11. Massie B, Conway M, Rajagopalan B, et al. Skeletal muscle metabolism during exercise under ischemic conditions in congestive heart failure. Evidence for abnormalities unrelated to blood flow. Circulation 1988;78:320-326.
12. Hill A, Lupton H. Muscular exercise, lactic acid and the supply and utilization of oxygen. Q J Med 1923;16:135-171.
13. Cerretelli P, Sikand R, Farhi L. Readjustment of cardiac output and gas exchange during onset of exercise and recovery. J Appl Physiol 1966;21:1355-1360.

14. Di Prampero P, Davies C, Cerretelli P, Maragaria R. An analysis of the oxygen debt contracted in submaximal exercise. J Appl Physiol 1970;29:547-551.

15. Henry F. Aerobic oxygen consumption and alactic debt in muscular work. J Appl Physiol 1951;3:427-438.

16. Hagberg J, Mullin J, Nagle F. Effect of work intensity and duration on recovery O_2. J Appl Physiol 1980;48:540-544.

17. Armon Y, Cooper D, Flores R, Zanconato S, Barstow T. Oxygen uptake dynamics during high intensity exercise in children and adults. J Appl Physiol 1991;70:841-848.

18. Massie B, Conway M, Yonge R, et al. 31P nuclear magnetic resonance evidence of abnormal skeletal muscle metabolism in patients with congestive heart failure. Am J Cardiol 1987;60:309-315.

19. Mancini D, Ferraro N, Tuchler M, Chance B, Wilson J. Detection of abnormal calf muscle metabolism in patients with heart failure using phosphorus-31 nuclear magnetic resonance. Am J Cardiol 1988;62:1234-1240.

20. Chati Z, Zannad F, Robin-Lherbier B, et al. Contribution of specific skeletal metabolic abnormalities to limitation of exercise capacity in patients with chronic heart failure: a 31P nuclear magnetic resonance study. Am Heart J 1994;128:781-792.

21. McCully K, Vandenborne K, DeMeirleir K, Posner J, Leigh JJ. Muscle metabolism in track athletes, using 31P magnetic resonance spectroscopy. Can J Physiol Pharmacol 1992;70:1353-1359.

22. Barstow T, Molé P. Simulation of pulmonary O_2 uptake during exercise transients in humans. J Appl Physiol 1987;63:2253-2261.

23. Barstow T, Lamarra J, Whipp B. Modulation of muscle and pulmonary O_2 uptakes by circulatory dynamics during exercise. J Appl Physiol 1990;66:979-989.

24. Belardinelli R, Barstow T, Nguyen P, Wasserman K. Skeletal muscle oxygenation and oxygen uptake kinetics following constant work rate exercise in chronic congestive heart failure. Am J Cardiol 1997;80:1319-1324.

25. Whipp B, Wasserman K. Oxygen uptake kinetics for various intensities of constant load work. J Appl Physiol 1972;33:351-356.

26. Girandola R, Katch F. Effects of physical conditioning on changes in exercise and recovery O_2 uptake and efficiency during constant-load ergometer exercise. Med Sci Sports Exerc 1973;5:242-247.

27. Hagberg J, Hickson R, Ehsani A, Holloszy J. Faster adjustment to and recovery from submaximal exercise in the trained state. J Appl Physiol 1980;48:218-224.

28. Convertino V, Goldwater D, Sandder H. $\dot{V}O_2$ kinetics of constant-load exercise following bed-rest-induced deconditioning. J Appl Physiol 1984;57:1545-1550.

29. Hughson R. Alterations in the oxygen deficit-oxygen debt relationships with beta-adrenergic receptor blockade in man. J Physiol 1984;349:375-387.

30. Chick T, Cagle T, Vegas F, Poliner J, Murata G. Recovery of gas exchange variables and heart rate after maximal exercise in COPD. Chest 1990;97:276-279.

31. Lim HY, Lee CW, Park SW, et al. Effects of percutaneous balloon mitral valvuloplasty and exercise training on the kinetics of recovery oxygen consumption after exercise in patients with mitral stenosis. Eur Heart J 1998;19:1865-1871.

32. de Groote P, Millaire A, Decoulx E, Nugue O, Guimier P, Ducloux G. Kinetics of oxygen consumption during and after exercise in patients with dilated cardiomyopathy: new markers of exercise intolerance with clinical implications. J Am Coll Cardiol 1996;28:168-175.

33. Tabet J, Logeart D, Bourgoin P, Guiti C, Alonso C, Cohen-Solal A. Prognostic value of "circulatory" power during exercise in patients with heart failure. J Am Coll Cardiol 2000;35(suppl A):181A. Abstract.

34. Osada N, Chaitman B, Miller L, et al. Cardiopulmonary exercise testing identifies low risk patients with heart failure and severely impaired exercise capacity considered for heart transplantation. J Am Coll Cardiol 1998;31:577-582.

35. Roul G, Moulichon M, Bareiss P, et al. Prognostic factors of chronic heart failure in NYHA class II or III: value of invasive exercise haemodynamic data. Eur Heart J 1995;16:1387-1398.

36. Mancini D, Katz S, Donchez L, Aaronson K. Coupling of hemodynamic measurements with oxygen consumption during exercise does not improve risk stratification in patients with heart failure. Circulation 1996;94:2492-2496.

37. Metra M, Faggiano P, D'Aloia A, et al. Use of cardiopulmonary exercise testing with hemodynamic monitoring in the prognostic assessment of ambulatory patients with chronic heart failure. J Am Coll Cardiol 1999;33:943-950.

38. Lauer MS, Okin PM, Larson MG, Evans JC, Levy D. Impaired heart rate response to graded exercise: prognostic implications of chronotropic incompetence in the Framingham Heart Study. Circulation 1996;93:1520-1526.

39. Cohen-Solal A, Czitrom D, Geneves M, Gourgon R. Delayed attainment of peak oxygen consumption after the end of exercise in patients with chronic heart failure. Int J Cardiol 1997;60:23-29.

40. Kremsen C, O'Toole M, Leff A. Oscillatory hyperventilation in severe congestive heart failure secondary to idiopathic dilated cardiomyopathy or to ischemic cardiomyopathy. Am J Cardiol 1987;59:900-905.

41. Feld H, Priest S. A cyclic breathing pattern in patients with poor left ventricular function and compensated heart failure: a mild form of Cheyne-Stokes respiration? J Am Coll Cardiol 1993;21:971-974.

42. Ribeiro J, Knutzen A, Rocco M, Hartley L, Colucci W. Periodic breathing during exercise in severe heart failure. Reversal with milrinone or cardiac transplantation. Chest 1987;92:555-556.

43. Yajima T, Koike A, Sugimoto K, Miyahara Y, Marumo F, Hiroe M. Mechanism of periodic breathing in patients with cardiovascular disease. Chest 1994;106:142-146.

44. Ben-Dov I, Sietsema KE, Casaburi R, Wasserman K. Evidence that circulatory oscillations accompany ventilatory oscillations during exercise in patients with heart failure. Am Rev Respir Dis 1992;145(4 Pt. 1):776-781.

45. Mortara A, Sleight P, Pinna GD, et al. Association between hemodynamic impairment and Cheyne-Stokes respiration and periodic breathing in chronic stable congestive heart failure secondary to ischemic or idiopathic dilated cardiomyopathy. Am J Cardiol 1999;84:900-904.

46. Ponikowski P, Anker S, Chua T, et al. Oscillatory breathing patterns during wakefulness in patients with chronic heart failure. Clinical implications and role of augmented peripheral chemosensitivity. Circulation 1999;100:2418-2424.

47. Chua TP, Clark AL, Amadi AA, Coats AJS. Relation between chemosensitivity and the ventilatory response to exercise in chronic heart failure. J Am Coll Cardiol 1996;27:650-657.

48. Francis D, Davies L, Piepoli M, Rauchlaus M, Ponikowski P, Coats A. Origin of oscillatory kinetics of respiratory gas exchange in chronic heart failure. Circulation 1999;100:1065-1070.

49. Andreas S, Hagenah G, Moller C, Werner GS, Kreuzer H. Cheyne-Stokes respiration and prognosis in congestive heart failure. Am J Cardiol 1996;78:1260-1264.

7

Time Constant for $\dot{V}O_2$ and Other Parameters of Cardiac Function in Heart Failure

Akira Koike, MD, Michiaki Hiroe, MD, and Haruki Itoh, MD

A symptom-limited incremental exercise test with the measurement of expired gas analysis is widely performed for evaluating exercise capacity in cardiac patients and for stratifying patients with heart failure.[1-8] Among indices of cardiopulmonary exercise testing, the peak O_2 uptake (peak $\dot{V}O_2$) measured at maximal exercise has been considered a "gold standard" because it reflects maximal cardiac output[5,7,8]; however, among cardiologists there is a considerable interest in obtaining objective information based on submaximal rather than maximal exercise.[4,9-12]

The increase in O_2 transport to muscle cells during the onset of exercise depends on circulatory function and is reflected in muscular $\dot{V}O_2$ kinetics. Thus, analysis of the kinetics of pulmonary $\dot{V}O_2$ during the onset of exercise, a parameter which closely reflects muscular $\dot{V}O_2$ kinetics, provides useful information on circulatory function in patients with cardiovascular disease.[13]

This chapter focuses on the clinical significance of parameters obtained during cardiopulmonary exercise testing, particularly the $\dot{V}O_2$ kinetics during constant work rate exercise, in patients with a variety of cardiovascular diseases.

Characteristics of $\dot{V}O_2$ Kinetics

The $\dot{V}O_2$ response during constant work rate exercise is postulated to have three phases[14,15]: phase I, an immediate increase at the start of exercise

This work was supported in part by a Grant-in-Aid for Scientific Research from the Ministry of Education, Science, and Culture of Japan.

From Wasserman K (ed): *Cardiopulmonary Exercise Testing and Cardiovascular Health.* Armonk, NY: Futura Publishing Company, Inc.; © 2002.

lasting approximately 20 seconds; phase II, a subsequent exponential increase that lasts 2 to 3 minutes; and phase III, a steady state level or slow drift phase that starts at approximately 3 minutes. If the exercise at a constant work rate is mild to moderate, $\dot{V}O_2$ usually reaches a steady state within 3 minutes.[13-15] At work rates associated with increased blood lactate, $\dot{V}O_2$ continues to increase beyond 3 minutes.[16-18] Thus, for the mild-intensity constant work rate exercise, the overall kinetics of $\dot{V}O_2$ can be determined objectively in terms of the time constant by fitting an exponential model to the increase of $\dot{V}O_2$.[13,14,18-20]

Figure 1 shows the $\dot{V}O_2$ response during and recovery from 50-W constant work rate exercise in a normal subject. After the onset of exercise, $\dot{V}O_2$ increases exponentially, and a single exponential equation fits well to the response of $\dot{V}O_2$. Longer time constant indicates slower kinetics of $\dot{V}O_2$ response. Thus, for the following studies, the time constant of $\dot{V}O_2$ kinetics was determined by fitting a single exponential function to the response starting at the onset of exercise, with the resting $\dot{V}O_2$ defined as the baseline, using the following equation:

$$\dot{V}O_2(t) = \dot{V}O_2(b) + A(1 - e^{-t/\tau}),$$

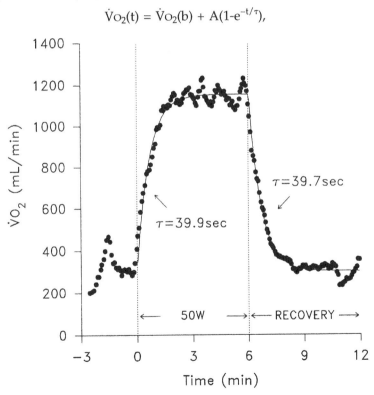

Figure 1. Changes in $\dot{V}O_2$ during 50 W of constant work rate exercise and during recovery, along with the computer-derived line of the best fit to a single exponential model of the $\dot{V}O_2$ response, for a normal subject. τ indicates time constant of $\dot{V}O_2$. Reproduced from reference 14 with permission.

where $\dot{V}_{O_2}$ (t) is $\dot{V}_{O_2}$ at time t, $\dot{V}_{O_2}$ (b) is the baseline $\dot{V}_{O_2}$ at rest, A is the amplitude of the $\dot{V}_{O_2}$ response (increment above baseline), and τ is the time constant. The time constant (τ) and amplitude (A) were derived by nonlinear regression analysis using least-squares and iterative techniques.[13,14,18,20] The time constant of $\dot{V}_{O_2}$ during recovery after exercise was determined similarly.

Relation Between $\dot{V}_{O_2}$ Kinetics and Cardiac Function During Exercise

During exercise, the increase in O_2 demand by muscle cells requires that their blood flow be increased. Thus, the increase in muscular $\dot{V}_{O_2}$ reflects the ability of O_2 supply to increase appropriately to meet the O_2 requirement, and is reflected in pulmonary $\dot{V}_{O_2}$.[21] Little is known, however, about the relation between resting cardiac function and kinetics of $\dot{V}_{O_2}$ in patients with cardiovascular disease.

To test the hypothesis that a small impairment in resting cardiac function can profoundly affect early dynamics of $\dot{V}_{O_2}$ and cardiac output during exercise, we measured both $\dot{V}_{O_2}$ and cardiac output during constant work rate exercise in 40 patients with myocardial infarction.[13] All the patients performed 6 minutes of mild-intensity constant work rate exercise (40 ± 8 W) using an upright bicycle ergometer. The exercise intensity was determined to correspond to 80% of the anaerobic threshold for each subject. Breath-by-breath $\dot{V}_{O_2}$ was measured throughout the test. Cardiac output was measured every 10 seconds using a radioisotope technique. The time constants of $\dot{V}_{O_2}$ and cardiac output were determined by fitting a single exponential function to each response. These time constants were compared after the subjects were divided into two groups; group 1 with the resting left ventricular ejection fraction (LVEF)$\geq$35% and group 2 with the LVEF<35%.

It was found that the time constant of $\dot{V}_{O_2}$ during constant work rate exercise was significantly longer (the kinetics were slower) in group 2 (58.0 ± 7.6 seconds) as compared to group 1 (45.8 ± 10.5 seconds, p=0.0002, Fig. 2). Although heart rate during exercise was consistently higher in group 2 than in group 1, the kinetics of the increase in heart rate in group 2 were also significantly slower (74.0 ± 30.9 vs. 47.8 ± 20.5 seconds, p=0.007). On the other hand, stroke volume in group 2 was lower throughout the exercise period.

Figure 3 demonstrates the response of cardiac output during the onset of exercise, determined by the changes in heart rate and stroke volume. There was no statistical difference in the resting cardiac output or cardiac output at the end of exercise between the two groups; however, the time constant of cardiac output was significantly slower in the patients with lower LVEF (63.0 ± 12.8 vs. 50.0 ± 12.2 seconds, p=0.005).

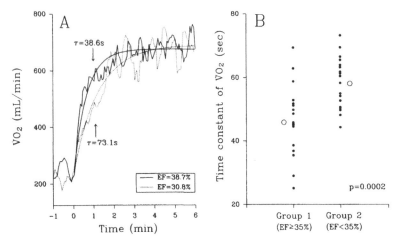

Figure 2. A. Computer-derived line of the best fit to a single exponential model of the V̇O₂ response in 2 patients: a patient with a left ventricular ejection fraction (EF) of 38.7% and a patient with EF of 30.8%. Both patients performed constant work rate exercise of 35 W (6 minutes). The V̇O₂ kinetics time constant (τ) was longer (the kinetics were slowed) in the patient with the lower EF. **B.** V̇O₂ response time constant for patients within the study. Open circles represent mean values. In group 1, the EF was ≥35%; in group 2, it was <35%. P value was determined by unpaired *t*-test. Reproduced from reference 13 with permission.

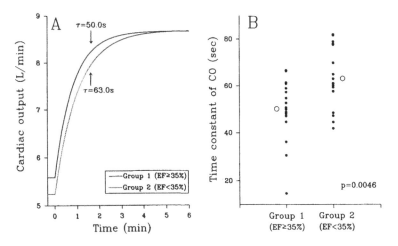

Figure 3. A. Mean change in cardiac output as related to time of group 1 (left ventricular ejection fraction [LVEF]≥35%) and group 2 (LVEF <35%) during constant work rate exercise. There was no statistical difference in the resting cardiac output and the cardiac output at 6 minutes of exercise between the 2 groups; however, the cardiac output time constant (τ) during exercise was longer in patients with lower ejection fractions (EF). **B.** The cardiac output (CO) time constant during constant work rate exercise in all patients. Open circles represent mean values. P value was determined by unpaired *t* test. Reproduced from reference 13 with permission.

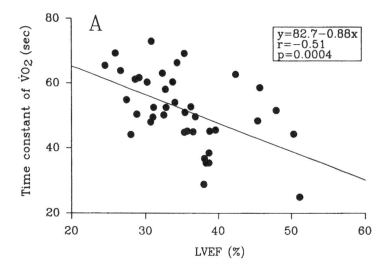

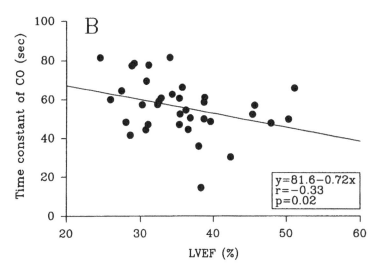

Figure 4. Relationship of the time constant of $\dot{V}O_2$ (**A**) and that of cardiac output (CO) (**B**) to resting left ventricular ejection fraction (LVEF). Reproduced from reference 13 with permission.

The relation between the resting LVEF and the time constants of $\dot{V}O_2$ and cardiac output is shown in Figure 4. The time constant of $\dot{V}O_2$ and that of cardiac output both significantly and negatively correlated with LVEF. Patients with lower LVEF had slower kinetics of $\dot{V}O_2$ and cardiac output. $\dot{V}O_2$ is determined by cardiac output (heart rate × stroke volume) and the difference in arterial and mixed venous O_2 content. Thus, a weak but significant correlation was noted between the time constant of cardiac output and that of $\dot{V}O_2$ ($r=0.30$, $p<0.05$) in these patients.

Relation Between $\dot{V}O_2$ Kinetics and Maximal Exercise Capacity

Since the $\dot{V}O_2$ kinetics during the onset of exercise are influenced profoundly by the response of cardiac function, it can be expected that the $\dot{V}O_2$ time constant is correlated with the parameters obtained during maximal exercise testing. We evaluated whether a decrease in maximal exercise capacity can be estimated by measuring $\dot{V}O_2$ kinetics during submaximal constant work rate exercise.[14]

The time constant of $\dot{V}O_2$ during the onset of exercise and the parameters of exercise capacity were measured in 14 normal subjects and 34 patients with cardiovascular disease. Their diagnoses were coronary artery disease (n=20), valvular heart disease (n=6), dilated cardiomyopathy (n=5), and the other heart disease (n=3). Each subject performed 50-W constant work rate exercise for 6 minutes and an incremental exercise test to the symptom-limited maximum using a cycle ergometer. From the constant work rate test, we determined the time constants of $\dot{V}O_2$ during exercise and recovery from exercise, using a single exponential equation.

The time constant of $\dot{V}O_2$ during 50-W constant work rate exercise showed a significant negative correlation with peak $\dot{V}O_2$ (r=−0.67, Fig. 5). The time constant was longer in the subjects with decreased peak $\dot{V}O_2$. There was a significant negative correlation between the time constant of $\dot{V}O_2$ and the maximal work rate obtained during a symptom-limited incremental exercise test (r=−0.66). The time constant of $\dot{V}O_2$ obtained during recovery from exercise also showed significant negative correlations with peak $\dot{V}O_2$ (r=−0.63) and maximal work rate (r=−0.54).

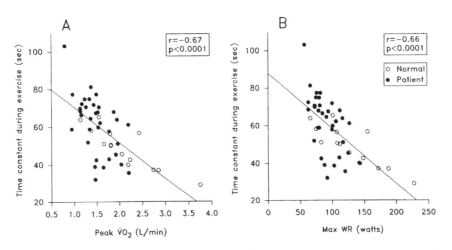

Figure 5. Relationship of the time constant of $\dot{V}O_2$ during 50 W of exercise to peak $\dot{V}O_2$ (**A**) and maximal work rate (**B**) obtained during the incremental exercise tests. Reproduced from reference 14 with permission.

Improvement of $\dot{V}O_2$ Kinetics by Coronary Vasodilators

On the basis of the above findings, we hypothesized that coronary vasodilators might speed the kinetics of the $\dot{V}O_2$ response at the onset of exercise by reducing myocardial ischemia and thereby improving cardiac function. In order to test this hypothesis, 10 patients with significant coronary stenosis performed mild-intensity constant work rate exercise (32 ± 3 W) for 6 minutes after oral administration of 10 mg of nicorandil (2-nicotinamidoethyl nitrate) or an identical placebo in a double-blind, crossover manner.[22] Nicorandil is a newly developed antianginal drug with potent vasodilating and antispastic properties.[23-26] As shown in Figure 6, the time constant for the increase in $\dot{V}O_2$ during constant work rate exercise, which characterizes the kinetics of $\dot{V}O_2$, was found to be significantly shorter after administration of nicorandil than after placebo (46.5 ± 13.3 vs. 51.1 ± 11.9 seconds; p=0.039). The increase in $\dot{V}O_2$ at 6 minutes compared with 3 minutes of constant work, which also reflects the $\dot{V}O_2$ kinetics, was reduced with nicorandil (3.8 ± 37.9 vs. 27.5 ± 27.1 mL/min; p=0.022).

Similarly, the effects of isosorbide dinitrate on the $\dot{V}O_2$ kinetics during the onset of mild-intensity constant work rate exercise (45 ± 13 W) were evaluated in 14 patients with significant coronary artery disease.[27] The time constant of $\dot{V}O_2$ was 44.5 ± 10.5 seconds after administration of a placebo (Fig. 7); however, it was shortened to 39.4 ± 10.1 seconds after administration of isosorbide dinitrate (p=0.038).

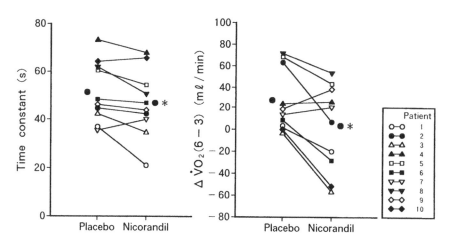

Figure 6. Effects of nicorandil on the time constant of $\dot{V}O_2$ and the increase in $\dot{V}O_2$ at 6 minutes as compared to 3 minutes [$\Delta\dot{V}O_2$ (6 − 3)] during exercise. Large closed circles represent mean values. *p=0.039 for the time constant of $\dot{V}O_2$ and 0.022 for $\Delta\dot{V}O_2$ (6−3) (paired t-test). Reproduced from reference 22 with permission.

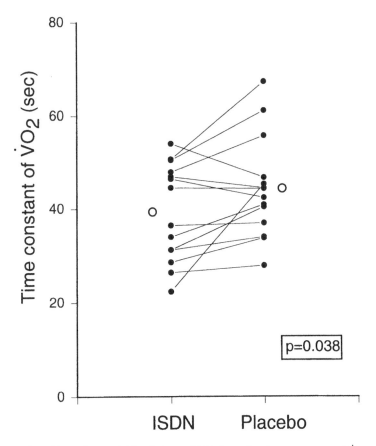

Figure 7. The effect of isosorbide dinitrate (ISDN) on the time constant of $\dot{V}O_2$ during constant work rate exercise. Reproduced from reference 27 with permission.

Improvement of $\dot{V}O_2$ Kinetics by Percutaneous Coronary Intervention

Although percutaneous coronary intervention (PCI) can be relied on to improve maximal exercise capacity by reducing myocardial ischemia and raising the threshold of the onset of anginal pain, it also may speed the kinetics of the cardiac output increase during exercise. An improved rise in cardiac output can be expected to speed the $\dot{V}O_2$ kinetics during exercise. Thus, we evaluated 17 patients with coronary artery disease who received successful PCI.[28] These patients performed constant work rate exercise at 50 W for 6 minutes and a symptom-limited incremental exercise test both before and 4 months after PCI procedure. Coronary angiography performed 4 months after PCI revealed that 3 out of 17 patients had restenosis in the target segment of a coronary vessel.

In the patients who had restenosis in the coronary arteries, indices of exercise capacity, including the time constant, were not changed and, in some cases, even worsened after PCI (Fig. 8). In the patients without restenosis, however, the time constant of $\dot{V}O_2$ kinetics was significantly shortened from 57.4 ± 12.6 seconds before PCI to 48.2 ± 9.5 seconds after PCI (p=0.004), indicating improved kinetics of the $\dot{V}O_2$ response. Since $\dot{V}O_2$ is the product of cardiac output and the difference in the O_2 content of arterial and venous blood, the significant shortening of the $\dot{V}O_2$ time constant was attributed to either a faster increase in cardiac output or a more rapidly increasing arteriovenous O_2 difference at the onset of exercise. In these patients, the peak $\dot{V}O_2$, gas exchange (anaerobic) threshold, and maximal work rate were also significantly increased after they underwent PCI.

Prognostic Significance of $\dot{V}O_2$ Kinetics in Patients with Cardiovascular Disease

Although peak $\dot{V}O_2$ has been used as a gold standard for stratifying patients with heart failure and identifying those with poor prognosis,[5,7,8] the time constant of $\dot{V}O_2$ may also be useful for identifying patients with poor prognosis. We therefore evaluated the prognostic significance of the $\dot{V}O_2$ time constant in 260 patients with cardiovascular disease.[29] The patients performed 4 minutes of 20-W exercise followed by a symptom-limited incremental exercise test on a cycle ergometer. The time constant of $\dot{V}O_2$ was determined during 4 minutes of 20-W exercise using a single exponential equation (Fig. 9). The data on mortality were examined 10 years after the exercise testing.

Twenty-nine cardiovascular-related deaths occurred after 3361 ± 610 days of follow-up. Peak $\dot{V}O_2$ and the gas exchange threshold were both significantly lower in nonsurvivors than in survivors. The time constant of $\dot{V}O_2$ in nonsurvivors was 76.7 ± 43.3 seconds and was significantly prolonged compared to that of survivors (55.3 ± 30.6 seconds, p=0.001). Kaplan-Meier survival curves for 10 years of follow-up demonstrated a survival rate of 89.0% for patients with a $\dot{V}O_2$ time constant<80 seconds and 71.7% for those with a time constant$\geq$80 seconds, showing a significant difference in survival (p=0.0028, Fig. 10). The patients with longer time constant were found to have significantly worse prognosis.

Summary

The time constant of $\dot{V}O_2$ during submaximal constant work rate exercise reflected lower ejection fraction at rest and delayed cardiac output response during the onset of exercise in patients with left ventricular dysfunction. The time constants of $\dot{V}O_2$ during exercise and recovery from

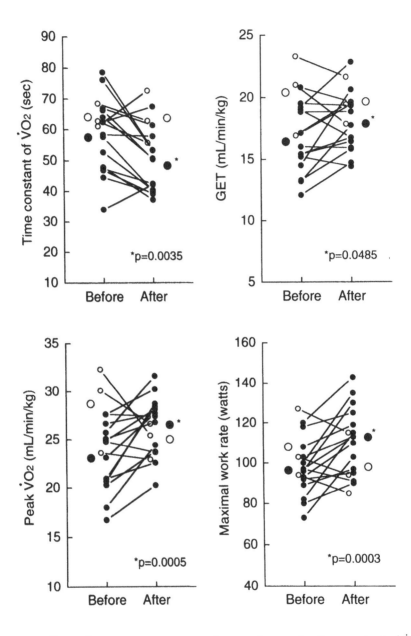

Figure 8. Effects of percutaneous coronary intervention on the time constant of V̇o₂, gas exchange (anaerobic) threshold (GET), peak V̇o₂, and maximal work rate in 14 patients without restenosis (closed circles) and 3 patients with restenosis (open circles). Large circles represent mean values. Reproduced from reference 28 with permission.

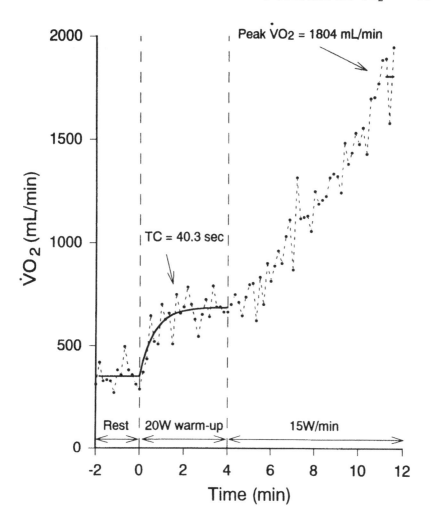

Figure 9. Changes in $\dot{V}O_2$ during 4 minutes of warm-up at 20 W followed by incremental exercise (1-W increase every 4 seconds) in a 45-year-old male patient with New York Heart Association functional Class I. The computer-derived line of the best fit to a single exponential model of the $\dot{V}O_2$ response during 20-W exercise is shown in a solid line. TC = time constant of $\dot{V}O_2$. Reproduced from reference 29 with permission.

exercise showed significant negative correlations with peak $\dot{V}O_2$ and maximal work rate. The time constant of $\dot{V}O_2$ was found to be a useful parameter for evaluating the effectiveness of therapy and for predicting long-term prognosis in patients with cardiovascular disease. We conclude that analysis of $\dot{V}O_2$ kinetics provides a useful parameter for the evaluation of circulatory adjustments at the onset of exercise in patients with cardiovascular disease and for identifying those with worse prognosis.

Survival Fraction

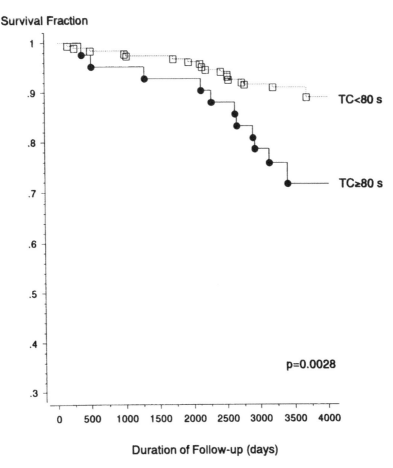

Figure 10. Kaplan-Meier survival curves for 10 years of follow-up showing a significant difference in survival between patients with a time constant (TC) of $\dot{V}O_2$ ≥80 seconds and those with a time constant <80 seconds (p=0.0028). Reproduced from reference 29 with permission.

References

1. Franciosa JA, Park M, Levine TB. Lack of correlation between exercise capacity and indexes of resting left ventricular performance in heart failure. Am J Cardiol 1981;47:33-39.
2. Weber KT, Janicki JS. Cardiopulmonary exercise testing for evaluation of chronic cardiac failure. Am J Cardiol 1985;55:22A-31A.
3. Wasserman K. New concepts in assessing cardiovascular function. Circulation 1988;78:1060-1071.
4. Itoh H, Koike A, Taniguchi K, Marumo F. Severity and pathophysiology of heart failure on the basis of anaerobic threshold (AT) and related parameters. Jpn Circ J 1989;53:146-154.

5. Mancini DM, Eisen H, Kussmaul W, Mull R, Edmunds LH, Wilson JR. Value of peak exercise oxygen consumption for optimal timing of cardiac transplantation in ambulatory patients with heart failure. Circulation 1991;83:778-786.

6. Cohn JN, Johnson GR, Shabetai R, et al. Ejection fraction, peak exercise oxygen consumption, cardiothoracic ratio, ventricular arrhythmias, and plasma norepinephrine as determinants of prognosis in heart failure. Circulation 1993;87(suppl VI):VI-5-VI-16.

7. Stelken AM, Younis LT, Jennison SH, et al. Prognostic value of cardiopulmonary exercise testing using percent achieved of predicted peak oxygen uptake for patients with ischemic and dilated cardiomyopathy. J Am Coll Cardiol 1996;27:345-352.

8. Opasich C, Pinna GD, Bobbio M, et al. Peak exercise oxygen consumption in chronic heart failure: toward efficient use in the individual patient. J Am Coll Cardiol 1998;31:766-775.

9. Sietsema KE, Cooper DM, Perloff JK, et al. Dynamics of oxygen uptake during exercise in adults with cyanotic congenital heart disease. Circulation 1986;73:1137-1144.

10. Koike A, Itoh H, Taniguchi K, Hiroe M. Detecting abnormalities in left ventricular function during exercise by respiratory measurement. Circulation 1989;80:1737-1746.

11. Sietsema KE, Ben-Dov I, Zhang YY, Sullivan C, Wasserman K. Dynamics of oxygen uptake for submaximal exercise and recovery in patients with chronic heart failure. Chest 1994;105:1693-1700.

12. Chua TP, Ponikowski P, Harrington D, et al. Clinical correlates and prognostic significance of the ventilatory response to exercise in chronic heart failure. J Am Coll Cardiol 1997;29:1585-1590.

13. Koike A, Hiroe M, Adachi H, et al. Oxygen uptake kinetics are determined by cardiac function at onset of exercise rather than peak exercise in patients with prior myocardial infarction. Circulation 1994;90:2324-2332.

14. Koike A, Yajima T, Adachi H, et al. Evaluation of exercise capacity using submaximal exercise at a constant work rate in patients with cardiovascular disease. Circulation 1995;91:1719-1724.

15. Wasserman K, Hansen JE, Sue DY, Whipp BJ, Casaburi R. Principles of Exercise Testing and Interpretation. Baltimore: Lippincott Williams & Wilkins; 1999:52-57.

16. Whipp BJ, Wasserman K. Oxygen uptake kinetics for various intensities of constant-load work. J Appl Physiol 1972;33:351-356.

17. Roston WL, Whipp BJ, Davis JA, Cunningham DA, Effros RM, Wasserman K. Oxygen uptake kinetics and lactate concentration during exercise in humans. Am Rev Respir Dis 1987;135:1080-1084.

18. Sietsema KE, Daly JA, Wasserman K. Early dynamics of O_2 uptake and heart rate as affected by exercise work rate. J Appl Physiol 1989;67:2535-2541.

19. Linnarsson D. Dynamics of pulmonary gas exchange and heart rate changes at start and end of exercise. Acta Physiol Scand (Suppl) 1974;415:1-68.

20. Koike A, Wasserman K, McKenzie DK, Zanconato S, Weiler-Ravell D. Evidence that diffusion limitation determines oxygen uptake kinetics during exercise in humans. J Clin Invest 1990;86:1698-1706.

21. Koike A, Wasserman K. Effect of acute reduction in oxygen transport on parameters of aerobic function during exercise. Ann Acad Med 1992;21:14-22.

22. Koike A, Hiroe M, Yajima T, et al. Effects of nicorandil on kinetics of oxygen uptake at the onset of exercise in patients with coronary artery disease. Am J Cardiol 1995;76:449-452.

23. Uchida Y, Yoshimoto N, Murao S. Effect of 2-nicotinamidethyl nitrate (SG-75) on coronary circulation. Jpn Heart J 1978;19:112-124.

24. Taira N, Satoh K, Yanagisawa T, Imai Y, Hiwatari M. Pharmacological profile of a new coronary vasodilator drug, 2-nicotinamidoethyl nitrate (SG-75). Clin Exp Pharmacol Physiol 1979;6:301-316.

25. Sakai K, Shiraki Y, Nabata H. Cardiovascular effects of a new coronary vasodilator N-(2-hydroxyethyl) nicotinamide nitrate (SG-75): comparison with nitroglycerin and diltiazem. J Cardiovasc Pharmacol 1981;3:139-150.

26. Hughes LO, Rose EL, Lahiri A, Raftery EB. Comparison of nicorandil and atenolol in stable angina pectoris. Am J Cardiol 1990;66:679-682.

27. Koike A, Yajima T, Koyama Y, et al. Effects of isosorbide dinitrate on oxygen uptake kinetics in cardiac patients. Med Sci Sports Exerc 1998;30:190-194.

28. Adachi H, Koike A, Niwa A, et al. Percutaneous transluminal coronary angioplasty improves oxygen uptake kinetics during the onset of exercise in patients with coronary artery disease. Chest 2000;118:329-335.

29. Koike A, Koyama Y, Itoh H, Adachi H, Marumo F, Hiroe M. Prognostic significance of cardiopulmonary exercise testing for 10-year survival in patients with mild to moderate heart failure. Jpn Circ J 2000;64:915-920.

8

Optimizing Decision Making in Heart Failure:

Applications of Cardiopulmonary Exercise Testing in Risk Stratification

Jonathan Myers, PhD

Despite important advances in therapy for patients with chronic heart failure (CHF), the mortality rate for this condition remains high and continues to be one of the important challenges facing clinicians who care for these patients. Cardiac transplantation has evolved into an important treatment option for patients with severe heart failure, but, because there continues to be a severe shortage of donor hearts, this option remains limited to a relatively small number of patients with end-stage disease. The high mortality rate and the widening gap between patients listed for transplantation and available donor hearts have magnified the need for reliable prognostic markers in CHF.

To direct the limited number of donor hearts to patients who need them the most, a great deal of effort has been directed toward stratifying risk among patients with severe CHF through the use of clinical, hemodynamic, and exercise test data. Consensus statements from the American Heart Association (AHA) and American College of Cardiology (ACC),[1,2] and a recent Bethesda Conference position statement[3] have helped establish guidelines for selection criteria among patients considered for transplantation (Table 1). In recent years, exercise capacity has been demonstrated to be a particularly important component of the risk profile among patients with CHF. During the last 10 years, at least 50 studies have demonstrated that peak O_2 uptake

From Wasserman K (ed): *Cardiopulmonary Exercise Testing and Cardiovascular Health.* Armonk, NY: Futura Publishing Company, Inc.; © 2002.

_____ Table 1 _____

Bethesda Conference Selection Criteria for Transplantation

I. Accepted indications for transplantation
  1. Peak $\dot{V}O_2$ <10 mL/kg/min with achievement of anaerobic metabolism
  2. Severe ischemia consistently limiting routine activity not amenable to bypass surgery or angioplasty
  3. Recurrent symptomatic ventricular arrhythmias refractory to all accepted therapeutic modalities
II. Probable indications for cardiac transplantation
  1. Peak $\dot{V}O_2$ <14 mL/kg/min and major limitation of the patient's daily activities
  2. Recurrent unstable ischemia not amenable to bypass or angioplasty
  3. Instability of fluid balance/renal function not due to patient noncompliance with regimen of weight monitoring, flexible use of diuretic drugs and salt restriction
III. Inadequate indications for Transplantation
  1. Ejection fraction
  2. History functional class III or IV symptoms of heart failure
  3. Previous ventricular arrhythmias
  4. Peak $\dot{V}O_2$ >15 mL/kg/min without other indications

From reference 3.

(peak $\dot{V}O_2$) is a significant univariate or multivariate predictor of outcomes in patients with CHF. Some of the larger studies are outlined in Table 2.[4-12]

Several important points can be made from the studies listed in Table 2 and others like them. First, peak $\dot{V}O_2$ has been demonstrated to be a significant predictor of outcomes in virtually every study performed among patients with CHF. Although previous studies have varied widely in terms of severity of heart failure, the use of different outcomes for assessing risk, application of different cut points for peak $\dot{V}O_2$, and inclusion or exclusion of other clinical, exercise, and hemodynamic variables, peak $\dot{V}O_2$ is clearly one of the more robust markers of risk in CHF. Directly measured peak $\dot{V}O_2$ in some studies has outperformed clinical, hemodynamic, and other exercise test data in predicting 1- to 2-year mortality.[4,8,12,13] Several investigators have reported that patients who achieve a peak $\dot{V}O_2 \geq 14$ mL/kg/min appear to have a prognosis similar to that among patients who receive transplantation (approximately 90% survival at 1 year). This finding implies that transplantation can be safely deferred among these patients. This cut point has emerged as a prominent prognostic marker in CHF and a value below this is listed as a relative indication for transplantation in the above mentioned guidelines.[1,3]

Questions that remain to be clarified include: 1) What is the place of cardiopulmonary exercise testing (CPET) relative to clinical, hemodynamic, and other data in the risk paradigm in patients with CHF? 2) What is the optimal cut point for peak $\dot{V}O_2$ when selecting patients for transplantation listing? 3) Should peak $\dot{V}O_2$ be expressed as an absolute value or corrected for age or body weight? 4) How well do other ventilatory gas exchange responses (e.g., the $\dot{V}E$ vs. $\dot{V}CO_2$ slope, gas exchange threshold, rate of recov-

Table 2

Summary of Some of the Major Studies Using Ventilatory Gas Exchange to Predict Outcomes in CHF

Author (ref#)	Study Type	Year	Subjects, n	Mean age, y	Mean Follow-up Period, mo	*Annual Mortality rate, %	Findings
Mancini et al.[4]	Prospective	1991	122	50±11	11±9	—	Peak $\dot{V}O_2$ >14 mL/kg/min had 6% first-year mortality vs. 53% in patients with peak $\dot{V}O_2$ ≤14 mL/kg/min
Stevenson et al.[8]	Prospective	1995	265	52±13	12	32	Peak $\dot{V}O_2$ ≤10 mL/kg/min was one of several predictors of death or urgent transplantation in patients with Class IV symptoms
Cohn et al.[7]	Prospective	1993	V-Heft I = 642; V-Heft II = 804	59.5±8	60	8	Peak $\dot{V}O_2$ was a highly significant univariate and multivariate predictor of survival
Saxon et al.[6]	Retrospective	1993	528	50±12	12±14	24	By univariate and multivariate analysis, peak $\dot{V}O_2$ <11 mL/kg/min was an independent predictor of heart failure death but not of sudden death.

Study	Design	Year	n				Comments
Chomsky et al.[11]	Prospective	1996	185	51.4±10	10±6	17	Peak $\dot{V}O_2$ (dichotomized at 10 mL/kg/min was an independent predictor of survival by univariate and multivariate analysis
Aaronson & Mancini[9]	Prospective	1995	272	52±12	24±18	33±3	Peak $\dot{V}O_2$ ≥14 mL/kg/min predicts survival; peak $\dot{V}O_2$ is a better predictor than % age-predicted $\dot{V}O_2$
Osada et al.[5]	Prospective	1998	500	50±10	25±17	15	Peak $\dot{V}O_2$ ≤14 mL/kg/min is a univariate and multivariate predictor of mortality; peak exercise SBP <120 mm Hg and % predicted peak $\dot{V}O_2$ ≤50% predicted mortality in patients with peak $\dot{V}O_2$ ≤14 mL/kg/min
Opasich et al.[10]	Prospective	1998	653	52±9	17±13	24	Peak $\dot{V}O_2$ stratified by <10, 10-18, and -mt18 mL/kg/min identified high, medium, and low risk
Myers et al.[12]	Retrospective	1998	644	48±11	47±28	5.3	Peak $\dot{V}O_2$ is a better predictor of survival than clinical, hemodynamic, or other exercise variables

CHF = chronic heart failure. *When not provided by investigator, number represents first-year mortality rate estimated from survival curve.

ery of $\dot{V}O_2$) predict risk? In this chapter, each of these issues is discussed in the context of risk stratification and decision making in patients with CHF.

Exercise Tolerance and Selection of Transplant Recipients

Because of the extreme shortage of donor hearts, recipients must be carefully selected to ensure optimal use of this scarce resource. In this regard, factors associated with 1- to 2-year survival among potential candidates are critical. Historically, the major factors associated with poor short-term outcome without transplantation have included an ejection fraction<15%, complex ventricular ectopy, sympathetic nervous system activation, and impaired exercise capacity, although there are many other clinical markers that have been associated with risk in CHF (Table 3). Moreover, selection criteria are in a state of change worldwide and there is variation in acceptance criteria from center to center. In addition, with recent advances in the treatment for CHF it has become apparent that for many patients once thought to have end-stage heart failure, the disease can be stabilized by aggressive medical therapy. Although predicting the clinical course in individual patients is imprecise, transplantation has been safely deferred in many patients by combinations of angiotensin-converting enzyme (ACE) inhibition or ACE-II blockade, diuretics, beta-blockade, and careful monitoring of patient status, including weight, electrolytes, and renal function. Other patients will deteriorate despite intensive medical management. Multidisciplinary heart failure

___ **Table 3** ___

Some of the Major Clinical Markers Associated with Risk in CHF

- Reduced ejection fraction
- Elevated pulmonary wedge pressure
- Reduced peak oxygen uptake
- Elevated catecholamine levels
- Reduced stroke work index
- Reduced cardiac output
- Reduced exercise capacity
- New York Heart Association functional class
- Reduced 6-minute walk performance
- Etiology of heart failure (coronary artery disease)
- Elevated plasma sodium
- Elevated plasma creatinine
- Presence of complex ventricular ectopy
- Inability to increase systolic blood pressure with exercise
- Reduced heart rate variability
- Duration of heart disease
- Male gender

CHF = chronic heart failure.

management programs have been set up to judiciously manage and monitor patients, and these programs have been shown to improve survival.[14] Most heart transplant centers have evolved into "heart failure management" clinics as well as facilities for transplantation.

Increased reliance on the role of exercise tolerance for decision making in CHF has occurred for several reasons. The recognition that exercise tolerance, expressed simply as workload achieved or exercise time, was a significant prognostic marker in patients with cardiovascular disease was made in the early 1970s.[15] Gas exchange techniques are now much more widespread, in part because of computerization and increased automation but also due to an appreciation for their applications to various cardiovascular and pulmonary disorders. In recent years, justification for their use in patients with CHF has been strengthened by a multitude of studies describing clinical applications of ventilatory and gas exchange abnormalities in CHF.[16] It is now common to use CPET as part of the standard work-up of the patient with CHF, and the available guidelines on transplantation consider this procedure an integral component among the indications for transplantation.[1-3] The widespread use of CPET in patients with CHF over the past 10 years has provided many groups the opportunity to evaluate the role of peak $\dot{V}O_2$ in prognosis.

Interaction Between Peak $\dot{V}O_2$ and Hemodynamic Variables in Stratifying Risk

Survival appears to be most accurately predicted when exercise variables are combined with clinical and hemodynamic data.[7,8,11,17-19] Historically, reduced left ventricular performance has been a common reason for referring a patient to a heart failure management clinic, and many studies have identified ejection fraction as a univariate or multivariate predictor of survival.[7,18,20,21] Ejection fraction by itself, however, is an inadequate reflection of left ventricular performance. Interestingly, it has been demonstrated that ejection fraction may lose its prognostic value in the very low range (i.e., <25%, the most clinically relevant range in patients considered for transplantation).[22] Conversely, others[7] have shown that ejection fraction engenders a marked increase in mortality once it is below 20%. Adding further confusion to this issue is the fact that ejection fraction and peak $\dot{V}O_2$ are poorly related.[23] Wilson et al.[24] recently observed that more than 50% of potential heart transplant candidates with reduced peak $\dot{V}O_2$ (mean 13.3±2.7 mL/kg/min) had only mild or moderate hemodynamic dysfunction during exercise, as evidenced by relatively normal increases in cardiac output and pulmonary wedge pressure. In the VHeFT studies,[7] ejection fraction and peak $\dot{V}O_2$ had an intriguing interaction; ejection fraction was more influential prognostically when peak $\dot{V}O_2$ was comparatively high (approximately twice as predictive when peak $\dot{V}O_2$ was >14.5 mL/kg/min).

Right heart catheterization is commonly performed in this population, to more directly assess cardiovascular performance and stratify risk. Variables such as low resting cardiac output and high intrapulmonary pressures have been associated with higher risk.[11,17,25,26] Some patients, however, remain markedly symptomatic despite normalization of cardiac output and left ventricular filling pressures. The level of exercise intolerance perceived by patients with heart failure has a questionable relation to objective measures of circulatory, ventilatory, or metabolic dysfunction during exercise.[24,27] In addition, these hemodynamic variables have not consistently been shown to be useful in prognosis.[4,8,12,28]

Nevertheless, peak $\dot{V}O_2$ has functioned synergistically with hemodynamic responses in some studies. Haywood et al.[17] observed that the combination of resting cardiac index and peak $\dot{V}O_2$ was 100% specific for identifying patients who could survive or avoid deterioration to "status one" (highest priority for transplantation) during the year after listing for heart transplantation. These investigators constructed tables based on a Cox proportional hazards model to predict the statistical chance of survival for any given cardiac index and peak $\dot{V}O_2$. Osada et al.[5] and the Stanford group[12] observed that the combination of peak $\dot{V}O_2$ and systolic blood pressure achieved during exercise increased the accuracy for predicting risk in patients evaluated for heart failure. It appears that the inability to increase systolic blood pressure beyond 120 to 130 mm Hg portends a higher risk.

Optimal Peak $\dot{V}O_2$ Cut Point for Stratifying Risk

The application of a single cut point for peak $\dot{V}O_2$ that can provide clinically meaningful separation between patients with high and low likelihood of survival is inherently attractive to clinicians because it greatly simplifies many of the complexities involved in predicting risk in CHF. In the mortality studies published during the last decade, it has been common to dichotomize patients above and below the median peak $\dot{V}O_2$ value for a given sample. A peak $\dot{V}O_2$ achieved that is lower than 14 mL/kg/min has been commonly applied in the context of selecting patients for transplantation, and is a relative indication for transplantation listing in the available guidelines.[1,3] However, many other cut points for peak $\dot{V}O_2$ have been advocated for stratifying risk in patients with CHF; differences between studies likely reflect differences in the severity of CHF in the different populations. A brief overview of some of the major studies follows.

In a landmark study that provided a springboard for many others, Mancini et al.[4] observed three groups of patients referred for transplantation for 2 years. One group comprised patients accepted for transplant on the basis of achieving a peak $\dot{V}O_2$ ≤14 mL/kg/min; a second group comprised patients considered too well for transplant (peak $\dot{V}O_2$ >14 mL/kg/min); and a third group comprised patients with a peak $\dot{V}O_2$ ≤14 mL/kg/min but who were rejected for transplantation for noncardiac reasons. Patients with preserved exercise capacity (>14 mL/kg/min) had 1- and 2-year survival rates of 94% and 84%, respectively, roughly equivalent to those observed after transplantation. This was contrasted by patients with poor exercise capacity (peak $\dot{V}O_2$ ≤14 mL/kg/min) who were rejected for transplantation, among whom 1- and 2- year survival rates were only 47% and 32%, respectively. By both univariate and multivariate analysis, peak $\dot{V}O_2$ was the best predictor of survival. This study has been widely cited as evidence that peak $\dot{V}O_2$ is an essential consideration when assessing a patient's suitability for transplant listing. Moreover, the study engendered the concept that a single cut point, 14 mL/kg/min, provides a clinically applicable cut point between patients who are likely to survive and those who are not.

Osada et al.[5] reported results from 500 patients observed for a mean of 25 months. Patients who achieved a peak $\dot{V}O_2$ >14 mL/kg/min had a 3-year survival rate of 93%, compared with 68% among patients whose peak $\dot{V}O_2$ was between 10 and 14 mL/kg/min. Patients whose peak $\dot{V}O_2$ was ≤14 mL/kg/min but >50% of their age- and gender-predicted value had a 3-year survival rate similar to that of patients who achieved a peak $\dot{V}O_2$ >14 mL/kg/min (93% vs. 91%). Patients with limited exercise capacity had a particularly poor survival if they were unable to raise peak exercise systolic blood pressure to at least 120 mm Hg; the 3-year survival rate among these patients was 55%, compared with an 83% survival rate among patients with a measurement ≤14 mL/kg/min whose peak exercise blood pressure was >120 mm Hg.

Roul et al.[29] prospectively studied 75 patients with clinical, radionuclide, and right heart catheterization data, and observed them for 1 year. The cohort was divided into two groups based on peak $\dot{V}O_2$ > or ≤14 mL/kg/min. Patients with preserved exercise capacity had lower left ventricular filling pressures, lower total peripheral resistance, lower creatinine and blood urea nitrogen levels, and higher exercise duration. During the 1-year follow-up, 9 patients died in the group with peak $\dot{V}O_2$ levels ≤14 mL/kg/min, whereas there were no deaths in the group with levels >14 mL/kg/min. Seven major events requiring hospitalization occurred in the limited exercise capacity group versus 3 in the preserved group.

Kao et al.[30] studied survival rates among 178 patients who underwent exercise testing at a baseline evaluation. Patients whose peak $\dot{V}O_2$ levels were <12 mL/kg/min had a higher mortality rate when compared to patients with peak $\dot{V}O_2$ levels >17 mL/kg/min. However, when patients were compared by tertiles of peak $\dot{V}O_2$ within the intermediate range (12 to 17 mL/kg/min), no differences in survival were observed between the tertiles. These investigators suggested that although peak $\dot{V}O_2$ differentiates patients who do and do not survive at the extremes of the exercise performance spectrum, the prognostic value of peak $\dot{V}O_2$ in the intermediate range (in which most patients fall) is limited.

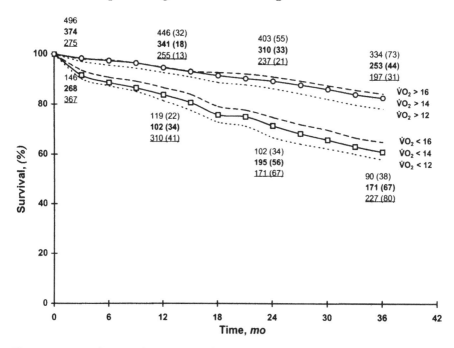

Figure 1. Survival curves for patients achieving above compared to below 12, 14, and 16 mL/kg/min for peak O_2 uptake. Numbers refer to patients evaluated at each time point for each survival curve; numbers in parentheses are cumulative numbers of deaths. From reference 12.

The Stanford data set of 644 patients with heart failure mentioned previously provided an ideal opportunity to assess the prognostic utility of 14 mL/kg/min and other cut points.[12] After 3 years of follow-up, patients who achieved levels >14 mL/kg/min had an 82% survival rate, whereas patients whose levels were ≤14 mL/kg/min had a 60% survival rate. Interestingly, this difference between survivors and nonsurvivors (approximately 20%) was similar when using any cut-off value between 10 and 17 mL/kg/min (Fig. 1). The survival curves were adjusted downward for the lower cut-off values and upward for the higher cut-off values, but one threshold did not appear to offer any advantage over another in terms of separating survivors from nonsurvivors.

Cardiopulmonary Markers of Risk Other than Peak $\dot{V}O_2$

Although peak $\dot{V}O_2$ defines the limits of the cardiopulmonary system, there are other cardiopulmonary responses that are important in defining the severity of CHF and prognosis. These responses are, to one extent or another, related to the ventilatory response to exercise, the capacity of the cardiopulmonary system to adapt to the demands of a given work rate, or the ability of the cardiopulmonary system to recover from a bout of exercise. In particular, there has recently been heightened interest in the $\dot{V}E$ vs. $\dot{V}CO_2$ slope below the point of ventilatory compensation for exercise lactic acidosis, as well as the kinetics of $\dot{V}O_2$ during recovery in risk stratification of patients with CHF.

The gas exchange threshold signaling the onset of the exercise lactic acidosis, one important submaximal marker of cardiopulmonary function with a long history, has been used in surprisingly few multivariate models to predict risk in CHF. Studies that have included the gas exchange threshold have demonstrated that $\dot{V}O_2$ at this point significantly predicts outcome. In the Stanford follow-up, $\dot{V}O_2$ at the gas exchange threshold was a significant univariate predictor of death in patients evaluated for CHF, but in a multivariate analysis peak $\dot{V}O_2$ was a stronger predictor of death.[12] This point has the potential to be a particularly useful marker of outcome since in many patients with CHF, "maximal" exercise is not achieved for various reasons or is difficult to define.

An impressive body of data has been published over the last several years demonstrating the role of the $\dot{V}E$ vs. $\dot{V}CO_2$ slope in predicting prognosis in CHF. This response is usually expressed as the slope of the best-fit linear regression line relating $\dot{V}E$ and $\dot{V}CO_2$ below the ventilatory compensation point for the exercise lactic acidosis. While the slope of this relationship is typically between 20 and 30 among normals, values in the 30s are common in patients with mild to moderate CHF, and values in the 40s are often observed in patients with more severe CHF.[31-34] In effect, a heightened $\dot{V}E$ vs. $\dot{V}CO_2$ slope is a reflection of the various physiological factors that underlie the abnormal ventilatory response to exercise in CHF.[35,36]

Models expressing the kinetics of $\dot{V}O_2$ at both exercise onset[37] and in recovery from exercise[38] have been used as prognostic markers in CHF. In a small series of patients, $\dot{V}O_2$ kinetics at exercise onset, expressed as a mean response time ≥60 seconds to a standardized protocol, was a stronger predictor of survival than peak $\dot{V}O_2$, the $\dot{V}E$ vs. $\dot{V}CO_2$ slope, and a variety of clinical and laboratory markers known to be related to CHF mortality.[37]

de Groote et al.[38] recently measured the ratio between total $\dot{V}O_2$ during exercise and recovery, the half-time of recovery of peak $\dot{V}O_2$, and the time constant of recovery in 153 patients with dilated cardiomyopathy. After a mean follow-up period of 15 months, the ratio of total $\dot{V}O_2$ during exercise and recovery was an independent predictor of survival in a subgroup of patients with moderate exercise intolerance, although not for the group as a whole. Similarly, Scrutinio et al.[39] followed 196 patients for a mean of 18 months and found that the half-time for $\dot{V}O_2$ in recovery was a significant independent predictor of death. Although data in this area are relatively limited, indices of O_2 kinetics are easy to determine with current automated gas exchange technology, and offer promise as supplemental indices to more precisely stratify risk in patients with CHF. Again, since these measures can be derived when exercise is submaximal, they may be particularly useful in CHF patients who are unable to exercise maximally.

Commentary on the Use of CPET and Risk in CHF

Directly measured $\dot{V}O_2$ has an established place in predicting outcomes in patients with CHF. Over the last decade, peak $\dot{V}O_2$ has been demonstrated in more than 50 studies to be an independent marker for risk of death or other endpoints. Increased automation of gas exchange systems has made these data easier to obtain, and this objective information is replacing the former dependence on subjective measures of clinical and functional status. Peak $\dot{V}O_2$ is now a recognized criterion for selecting patients who could potentially benefit from heart transplantation.[1-4] It is often a more powerful predictor of death when combined with other clinical, hemodynamic, and exercise data.[6,7,12,17]

Clearly, however, there are several specific areas that require further study. A peak $\dot{V}O_2$ of 14 mL/kg/min is a widely used cut-off point to separate survivors from nonsurvivors, and therefore is commonly used to help select patients for transplantation. However, it is not entirely clear whether there is a specific cut point that optimally separates survivors from nonsurvivors. Studies have demonstrated that each peak $\dot{V}O_2$ value ranging from 10 to 17 mL/kg/min may represent an "optimal" cut-off point; more than likely, this value changes depending on the severity of heart failure in the population studied.

Peak $\dot{V}O_2$ is influenced by age, gender, body weight, and mode of exercise, and some studies have demonstrated that peak $\dot{V}O_2$ expressed as a percentage of the predicted value (taking these variables into account) is a more powerful predictor of outcome than absolute peak $\dot{V}O_2$ achieved.[5,40] However, previous studies are evenly split in regard to whether $\dot{V}O_2$ adjusted to percentage of normal outperforms absolute peak $\dot{V}O_2$. Two studies have suggested that the estimate of survival using percent of age-predicted $\dot{V}O_2$ is enhanced in women,[9,41] but this observation requires further study. One issue that complicates this approach is the fact that there are many age- and gender-predicted "standards" for peak $\dot{V}O_2$.[42]

The majority of studies have not been large enough to perform a valid assessment of mortality, perhaps because gas exchange techniques have not been widely used in this context until recently. In many of the studies performed in the 1980s, the number of endpoints was particularly low, and the ratio of independent (predictor) variables to the number of endpoints was inappropriate to address this question in a valid fashion. In many of the widely cited studies that examined subgroups (i.e., stratified by peak $\dot{V}O_2$ cut point, type of heart failure, gender, and so forth), there were less than 10 deaths in each of the specified subgroups. Moreover, in few of these studies were patients observed longer than a mean of 1 year. Only in recent years have studies been large enough (i.e., >500 in a cohort) or powerful enough (i.e., adequate numbers of deaths over long enough follow-up) to make confident conclusions in terms of predicting survival.

Relative to peak $\dot{V}_{O_2}$, hemodynamic variables are inconsistent in their ability to predict risk of death or clinical deterioration. The dissociation between hemodynamic observations and exercise responses[24,27] underscores the complex nature of heart failure. Exertional symptoms and hemodynamic variables should be treated as separate entities; the former is influenced by musculoskeletal metabolism and strength, body composition, and motivation, in addition to cardiac function, whereas the latter is influenced largely by the degree of pump dysfunction. Nevertheless, peak $\dot{V}_{O_2}$ is a more powerful predictor of risk when combined with one or more hemodynamic variables.[6,7,17]

Comparing or summarizing studies that have used different outcomes is also problematic. Many of the studies discussed in this chapter have used, in addition to deaths, softer endpoints such as hospitalizations, transplantation, change in listing status for transplantation, and others. Although this is often done to increase the number of study endpoints, such a study can no longer be considered one of "survival," and the subjectivity of many of these endpoints introduces the potential for significant bias and other errors that reduce the confidence in the study results. Although endpoints other than death are important outcomes clinically, they generally should not be used in survival analysis, and transplantation should be a censored event because this procedure completely changes the natural course of treatment and the disease. Future studies should also make every effort to classify causes of death by sudden versus progressive heart failure or noncardiac. The latter has rarely been done in previous studies, yet it is an important distinction clinically if the cardiologist is to know whether an intervention to prevent a lethal arrhythmia or to improve pump function is the more reasonable therapeutic approach to a given patient.

Although it seems clear that peak $\dot{V}_{O_2}$ has a vital role in predicting risk in heart failure populations, it has also been demonstrated that, as in patients with coronary artery disease, maximal exercise duration also predicts risk in heart failure. Because maximal exercise time and peak $\dot{V}_{O_2}$ are correlated during exercise, some have suggested that these two variables could be used interchangeably when assessing exercise tolerance, and this raises the issue as to whether directly measured $\dot{V}_{O_2}$ offers any additional prognostic power over exercise time or workload achieved. This question is not a trivial one, because if exercise time has equivalent prognostic power, it would obviate the need for specialized laboratory equipment, time, expense, and patient discomfort associated with gas exchange analysis. Compared with exercise time or workload achieved, the direct cardiopulmonary response is not only more precise but offers a great deal of additional insight into the physiology of exercise intolerance.[16,42] Again, previous studies have generally not been large enough nor have data been gathered prospectively in a manner that would permit the comparison between measured and estimated $\dot{V}O_2$ in prognosis; only one study has performed such a comparison.[12] In that study, both peak $\dot{V}O_2$ and watts achieved on a cycle ergometer were significant univariate predictors of death, although measured peak $\dot{V}O_2$ was clearly a more important variable; by multivariate analysis it was the only predictor of death. Similar findings were implied in the study of Willens et al.[43] and the VHeFT data,[7] but the former study involved only 8 deaths (out of 30 patients over 15 months), and in the latter study the predictive power of exercise time was not presented, although it was stated that peak $\dot{V}O_2$ was a better predictor of survival.

Summary

It should be noted that a plethora of variables have been shown in various studies to predict outcome in patients with heart failure. There have been more than 150 clinical, hemodynamic, or exercise variables identified as predictors of mortality. Obviously, many are interrelated, and it is not possible to measure them all in a given study. This underscores that exercise capacity should not be the sole determinant in any risk stratification model or in transplant candidate selection. Assessment of risk in patients with heart failure remains largely an art form; any risk paradigm should be made in the context of a variety of prognostic markers. Several groups in the US with large transplant centers[5,8,12,28] are continuing to collect data prospectively, and answers to some of these difficult questions will no doubt be forthcoming as these and other data sets become larger and more robust.

References

1. O'Connell JB, Bourge RC, Costanzo-Nordin M, et al. Cardiac transplantation: recipient selection, donor procurement, and medical follow-up: a statement for health professionals from the Committee on Cardiac Transplantation of the Council on Clinical Cardiology. American Heart Association. Circulation 1992;86: 1061-1079.

2. Costanzo MR, Augustine S, Bourge R, et al. Selection and treatment of candidates for heart transplantation: a statement for health professionals from the Committee on Heart Failure and Cardiac Transplantation of the Council on Clinical Cardiology. American Heart Association. Circulation 1995;92:3593-3612.

3. Mudge GH, Goldstein S, Addonizio LJ, et al. Twenty-fourth Bethesda Conference: cardiac transplantation: Task Force 3: recipient guidelines/prioritization. J Am Coll Cardiol 1993;22:21-31.

4. Mancini DM, Eisen H, Kussmaul W, Mull R, Edmunds LH, Wilson JR. Value of peak exercise oxygen consumption for optimal timing of cardiac transplantation in ambulatory patients with heart failure. Circulation 1991;83:778-786.

5. Osada N, Chaitman BR, Miller LW, et al. Cardiopulmonary exercise testing identifies low risk patients with heart failure and severely impaired exercise capacity considered for heart transplantation. J Am Coll Cardiol 1998;31:577-582.

6. Saxon LA, Stevenson WG, Middlekauff HR, et al. Predicting death from progressive heart failure secondary to ischemic or idiopathic dilated cardiomyopathy. Am J Cardiol 1993;72:62-65.

7. Cohn JN, Johnson GR, Shabetai R, et al. Ejection fraction, peak exercise oxygen consumption, cardiothoracic ratio, ventricular arrhythmias, and plasma norepinephrine as determinants of prognosis in heart failure. Circulation 1993;87(suppl VI):VI-16.

8. Stevenson LW, Couper G, Natterson B, et al. Target heart failure populations for newer therapies. Circulation 1995;92(suppl II):II-174-II-181.

9. Aaronson KD, Mancini DM. Is percentage of predicted maximal exercise oxygen consumption a better predictor of survival than peak exercise oxygen consumption for patients with severe heart failure? J Heart Lung Transplant 1995;14: 981-989.

10. Opasich C, Pinna GD, Bobbio M, et al. Peak exercise oxygen consumption in chronic heart failure: toward efficient use in the individual patient. J Am Coll Cardiol 1998;31:766-775.

11. Chomsky DB, Lang CC, Rayos GH, et al. Hemodynamic exercise testing: a valuable tool in the selection of cardiac transplantation candidates. Circulation 1996;94:3176-3183.

12. Myers J, Gullestad L, Vagelos R, et al. Clinical, hemodynamic, and cardiopulmonary exercise test determinants of outcome in patients referred for evaluation of heart failure. Ann Intern Med 1998;129:286-293.

13. Myers J, Gullestad L. The role of exercise testing and gas exchange measurement in the prognostic assessment of patients with heart failure. Curr Opin Cardiol 1998;13:145-155.

14. Stewart S, Marley JE, Horowitz JD. Effects of a multidisciplinary, home-based intervention on planned readmissions and survival among patients with chronic congestive heart failure: a randomized controlled trial. Lancet 1999;354:1077-1083.

15. Ellestad MH, Wan MKC. Predictive implications of stress testing: follow-up of 1700 subjects after maximum treadmill stress testing. Circulation 1975;51:363.

16. Wasserman K, Hansen JE, Sue DY, Casaburi R, Whipp BJ. Principles of Exercise Testing and Interpretation. 3rd ed. Philadelphia: Lippincott, Williams & Wilkins; 1999.

17. Haywood GA, Rickenbacher PR, Trindade PT, et al. Analysis of deaths in patients awaiting heart transplantation: impact on patient selection criteria. Heart 1996;75:455-462.

18. Madsen BK, Hansen JF, Stokholm KH, Brons J, Husum D, Mortensen LS. Chronic congestive heart failure. Description and survival of 190 consecutive patients with a diagnosis of chronic congestive heart failure based on clinical signs and symptoms. Eur Heart J 1994;15:303-310.

19. Robbins M, Francis G, Pashkow FJ, et al. Ventilatory and heart rate responses to exercise: better predictors of heart failure mortality than peak oxygen consumption. Circulation 1999;100:2411-2417.

20. Likoff MJ, Chandler SL, Kay HR. Clinical determinants of mortality in chronic congestive heart failure secondary to idiopathic dilated or to ischemic cardiomyopathy. Am J Cardiol 1987;59:634-638.

21. Gradman A, Deedwania P, Cody R, et al., for the Captopril-Digoxin Study Group. Predictors of total mortality and sudden death in mild to moderate heart failure. J Am Coll Cardiol 1989;14:564-570.

22. Dec GW. Idiopathic dilated cardiomyopathy. N Engl J Med 1994;331:1564-1575.

23. Myers J, Froelicher VF. Hemodynamic determinants of exercise capacity in chronic heart failure. Ann Intern Med 1991;115:377-386.

24. Wilson JR, Rayos G, Keoh TK, Gothard P. Dissociation between peak exercise oxygen consumption and hemodynamic dysfunction in potential heart transplantation candidates. J Am Coll Cardiol 1995;26:429-435.

25. Francis GS. Determinants of prognosis in patients with heart failure. J Heart Lung Transplant 1994;12:S113-S116.

26. Unverferth DV, Magorien RD, Moeschberger ML, Baker PB, Fetters JK, Leier CV. Factors influencing the one-year mortality of dilated cardiomyopathy. Am J Cardiol 1984;54:147-152.

27. Wilson JR, Rayos G, Yeoh TK, Gothard P, Bak K. Dissociation between exertional symptoms and circulatory function in patients with heart failure. Circulation 1995;92:47-53.

28. Aaronson KD, Schwartz JS, Chen T-M, Wong K-L, Goin JE, Mancini DM. Development and prospective validation of a clinical index to predict survival in ambulatory patients referred for cardiac transplant evaluation. Circulation 1997;95:2660-2667.

29. Roul G, Moulichon M-E, Bareiss P, et al. Exercise peak $\dot{V}O_2$ determination in chronic heart failure: is it still of value? Eur Heart J 1994;15:495-502. 30. Kao W, Winkel EM, Johnson MR, Piccione W, Lichtenberg R, Constanzo MR. Role of maximal oxygen consumption in establishment of heart transplant candidacy for heart failure patients with intermediate exercise tolerance. Am J Cardiol 1997;79:1124-1127.

31. Wada O, Asanoi H, Miyagi K, et al. Importance of abnormal lung perfusion in excessive exercise ventilation in chronic heart failure. Am Heart J 1992;125: 790-798.

32. Kleber FX, Vietzke G, Wernecke KD, et al. Impairment of ventilatory efficiency in heart failure: prognostic impact. Circulation 2000;101:2803-2809.

33. Bol E, de Vries WR, Mosterd WL, Wielenga RP, Coats AJ. Cardiopulmonary exercise parameters in relation to all-cause mortality in patients with chronic heart failure. Int J Cardiol 2000;72:255-263.

34. Francis DP, Shamim W, Davies LC, et al. Cardiopulmonary exercise testing for prognosis in chronic heart failure: continuous and independent prognostic value from $\dot{V}E/\dot{V}CO_2$ slope and peak $\dot{V}O_2$. Eur Heart J 2000;21:154-161.

35. Sullivan MJ, Higginbotham MB, Cobb FR. Increased exercise ventilation in chronic heart failure: intact ventilatory control despite hemodynamic and pulmonary abnormalities. Circulation 1988;77:552-559.

36. Wasserman K, Zhang Y-Y, Gitt A, et al. Lung function and exercise gas exchange in chronic heart failure. Circulation 1997;96:2221-2227.

37. Brunner-La Rocca HP, Weilenman D, Schalcher C, et al. Prognostic significance of oxygen uptake kinetics during low level exercise in patients with heart failure. Am J Cardiol 1999;84:741-744.

38. de Groote P, Millaire A, Decoulx E, Nugue O, Guimier P, Ducloux G. Kinetics of oxygen consumption d*SO1*d*SO0*uring and after exercise in patients with dilated cardiomyopathy. J Am Coll Cardiol 1996;28:168-175.

39. Scrutinio D, Passantino A, Lagioia R, Napoli F, Ricci A, Rizzon P. Percent achieved of predicted peak exercise oxygen uptake and kinetics of recovery of oxygen uptake after exercise for risk stratification in chronic heart failure. Int J Cardiol 1998;64:117-124.

40. Stelken AM, Younis LT, Jennison SH, et al. Prognostic value of cardiopulmonary exercise testing using percent achieved of predicted peak oxygen uptake for

patients with ischemic and dilated cardiomyopathy. J Am Coll Cardiol 1996;27:345-352.

41. Richards DR, Mehra MR, Ventura HO, et al. Usefulness of peak oxygen consumption in predicting outcome of heart failure in women verses men. Am J Cardiol 1997;80:1236-1238.

42. Myers J. Essentials of Cardiopulmonary Exercise Testing. Champaign, IL: Human Kinetics Publishers; 1996.

43. Willens HJ, Blevins RD, Wrisley D, Antonishen D, Reinstein D, Rubenfire M. The prognostic value of functional capacity in patients with mild to moderate heart failure. Am Heart J 1987;114:377-382.

9

Preoperative Assessment of Elderly Surgical Patients

Paul Older, MB and Adrian Hall, MB

In the late 1970s and early 1980s, there was an explosion in the use of high technology in industry. Medicine, traditionally conservative, did not rapidly embrace this new "industrial revolution." Certainly in most hospitals at that time, the intensive care units (ICUs) relied more on clinical expertise than invasive measurements and high technology. The mid 1980s saw a large increase in the use of invasive monitoring systems in the treatment of critically ill patients. Much of the workload of ICUs at that time involved patients with postsurgical complications. The intensive care specialists, however, were not involved until late in the postoperative period when the patient had already deteriorated on the ward. Patients were only admitted to ICU when they were acutely ill with multisystem failure and a high APACHE score.[1] The delays in referral and definitive treatment resulted in a high mortality.[2] Furthermore, the duration of stay was excessively prolonged because of high morbidity. The latter was a major drain on intensive care resources and remains so today.

In 1960, Clowes and Del Guercio[3] demonstrated that perioperative mortality was related to poor ventricular function, but this work was clearly not known to a wide audience. Shoemaker[4] elaborated on this concept in 1972 by characterizing the differing physiological variables in surviving and non-surviving surgical patients. Goldman and Caldera[5] published their seminal article on clinical evaluation of cardiac risk in noncardiac surgical patients in 1977. Despite this information, throughout the 1970s the concept of risk identification and subsequent triage of patients to differing levels of perioperative management was not practiced. It was not until Professors Louis Del Guercio and Joseph Cohn[6] used pulmonary artery catheters to identify poor

From Wasserman K (ed): *Cardiopulmonary Exercise Testing and Cardiovascular Health.* Armonk, NY: Futura Publishing Company, Inc.; © 2002.

ventricular function preoperatively in 1980 that any concept of preoperative identification of risk based on physiological measurement was developed.

In 1988, our group published the results of preoperative assessment of physiological variables by pulmonary artery catheter.[7] This study was the genesis of our integrated approach to perioperative risk assessment and management. Before our study, the documented mortality rate at our hospital was 19%; this information was obtained from a retrospective analysis from 1980 to 1983 of major abdominal surgery in patients over 65 years. Postsurgical management at that time followed the model described above.

Over a period of 3 years, starting in 1984, we studied 100 elderly patients scheduled for major surgery. Using methods similar to those used by Del Guercio and colleagues, we used pulmonary artery catheters preoperatively, as a screening test, to identify patients at increased surgical risk. At that time, the pulmonary artery catheter had been in clinical use in Australia for only 6 years and was not widely used by intensive care physicians.

This 1984 study highlighted three major issues. First, mortality compared to the 3 preceding years had been improved from 19% to 6%. The only change was that the patients were managed perioperatively by intensive care specialists in an ICU. Second, 11% of the patients had severe ventricular dysfunction with a resting cardiac index of $<2.2 \text{ mL/min/M}^2$. Third, as no preoperative or postoperative problem was demonstrated in many of the patients who had been admitted to the ICU, an expensive resource was being wasted.

In 1987, the Confidential Enquiry into Perioperative Deaths (CEPOD)[8] was published and demonstrated in a series 500,000 patients that postoperative deaths occurred predominantly in patients over 70 years of age having major surgery with preexisting cardiac or pulmonary disease. Three main points need emphasis: elderly patients, major surgery, and preexisting disease. This is the same group of patients identified by Goldman and Caldera[5] in 1977. We saw the need for a better method of evaluation of surgical risk. We hypothesized that exercise gas exchange could be used to achieve this.

In 1988 we began to use cardiopulmonary exercise testing (CPET) to look for preexisting cardiac and pulmonary disease preoperatively on a routine basis. The major consideration was that it was to be used as a tool for the routine evaluation of all elderly patients scheduled for major surgery, i.e., as a screening test. We suspected that cardiopulmonary disease exists in an occult state in the elderly. If the test was restricted to those with clinically detectable heart disease, then 'occult' disease would be missed and we would miss the very group we were trying to identify.

The increase in O_2 uptake ($\dot{V}O_2$) under exercise conditions, as a concept, was not new; it had been understood since the late 1700s. Antoine Laurent Lavoisier, the man who named 'oxygen,' demonstrated the increase in air consumption of a subject lifting a 15-pound weight an accumulated height of 600 feet in 15 minutes. In May 1794 he went to the guillotine for his work: "the revolution has no need of scientists." [*Editor's note: Perkins' brief but superb account of Lavoisier's remarkable contributions to the science of his day describes more precisely the circumstances that led to his execution. Lavoisier was one of 60 members of an organization in France that functioned as the King's "Internal Revenue Service." Thus, Lavoisier was authorized to collect taxes on behalf of the King from the people, and being allowed a profit in doing so. It was from these funds that he was able to buy his costly equipment. Perkins notes that while he was not abusive in this authority, in contrast to some of his predecessors, it was this charge that led Lavoisier to his death by the guillotine. (Perkins JF Jr. Historical development of respiratory physiology. In Fenn WO, Rahn H (eds): Handbook of Physiology. Sec. 3. Respiration. Vol. 1. Washington, DC: Am Physiol Soc. 1964:1-62)].*

The direct measurement of $\dot{V}O_2$ as a noninvasive clinical procedure had to wait for the development of commercial metabolic carts that became available in the early 1980s. Under conditions of exercise, $\dot{V}O_2$ increase is proportional to cardiac output. Using a metabolic cart, it is easy to evaluate cardiac and pulmonary performance during exercise by measurement of $\dot{V}O_2$ and other parameters of respiratory gas exchange. This is the basis of CPET. As it is noninvasive, inexpensive to perform, and may be performed on outpatients, it offered us the ideal method of screening patients for cardiopulmonary risk assessment. Such testing need not be to maximum exercise capacity but may be stopped shortly after the anaerobic threshold (*AT*) is reached. This point is easy to detect during the test and is a volitionally independent marker of sustainable aerobic function.

Assessment of Cardiac Risk for Noncardiac Surgery

Age is not a predictor of individual risk. In terms of group statistics, *AT* decreases with advancing age (Fig. 1), but one standard deviation embraces the population from the age of 55 years to 85 years. Wasserman[9] pointed out that we age at different rates and therefore the use of age as a discriminator will result in fit elderly patients being denied life-saving surgery while allowing a younger patient with occult cardiovascular disease to proceed to surgery, only to succumb to it.

Clinical assessment of risk will detect a large group of patients with overt cardiopulmonary disorders but can miss those with more occult disease. CPET will detect the group that such clinical examination will miss.

For many years, attention has focused preoperatively on detection of myocardial ischemia. Some published studies have made assumptions of myocardial ischemia on the basis of a history of risk factors[10,11] without any proof of the diagnosis. This approach is flawed from two perspectives. First, some patients who are asymptomatic and have no "risk factors" may have myocardial ischemia. Second, not all patients with risk factors have coronary artery disease. Other studies have not distinguished the type of surgery for

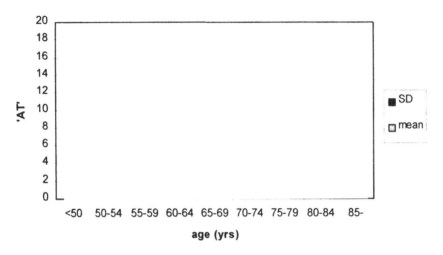

Figure 1. Effect of age on the anaerobic threshold (AT) in 675 patients.

which the patient is scheduled.[11] As is discussed later, this is an important issue. Little attention has been paid to issues of cardiac failure[12] and postoperative stress response, despite the earlier work of Goldman and Caldera,[5] Del Guercio, Cohn, and Clowes,[3,6] and Shoemaker.[4] We hypothesize that the major determinant of perioperative mortality is the inability of the heart to increase output to match the increase in oxygen demand mandated by major surgery and the postsurgical period. Myocardial ischemia may be a cause of cardiac failure or may be caused by an increase in myocardial oxygen demand resulting from an increase in cardiac output. In two published studies involving more than 700 elderly patients, we showed that mortality rate is correlated with cardiac failure.[13,14] Certainly the association of myocardial ischemia with cardiac failure increases the risk, but patients exhibiting myocardial ischemia in the absence of cardiac failure appear not to be at risk.

The American College of Cardiology/American Heart Association Guidelines

The American College of Cardiology/American Heart Association guidelines[15] is a consensus document published by a task force in 1996. The patient population is classified into three risk groups on the basis of cardiac risk: low, intermediate, and high. The low-risk group includes those under 60 years of age with no history of cardiopulmonary disease, while the high-risk group includes patients with acute coronary syndromes, decompensated cardiac failure, and supraventricular arrhythmias. There could be little argument about these groupings. The problem lies in the intermediate group, in which clinical indicators are unreliable, age is a poor discriminator, and occult cardiac failure and/or myocardial ischemia does occur. In our own studies some 25% of patients over 60 years of age have an *AT* below 11 mL/kg/min and 25% have silent myocardial ischemia.[13,14,16] While some patients fall into both groups, either pathology may exist independent of the other. It is this group of patients in whom CPET will reveal such problems. In our studies, myocardial ischemia was detected in only 35% of the patients at risk.[13]

The guidelines also introduce the important concept of 'surgery-specific risk.' This concept is based on the fact that minor surgery (e.g., peripheral surgery) is not associated with the large increase in oxygen demand of major intracavity surgery. We prefer to define surgery-specific risk in terms of postoperative increase in $\dot{V}O_2$. We classify low-risk surgery as that associated with a likely postoperative $\dot{V}O_2$ <120 mL/M^2, intermediate-risk surgery where the $\dot{V}O_2$ is likely to be between 120 and 150 mL/M^2, and high-risk surgery as that in which it is likely to be in excess of 150 mL/M^2. We have demonstrated the average $\dot{V}O_2$ following major intra-abdominal surgery as 170 mL/M^2.[7]

The guidelines endorse the use of maximal exercise capacity estimated as metabolic equivalents (METS). One MET is the $\dot{V}O_2$ of a resting 40-year-old, 70-kg male, and is approximately 3.5 mL/kg/min. While we agree in general terms with these guidelines, we feel that estimation of functional capacity in terms of METS leads to unacceptable inaccuracy. The guidelines suggest that patients unable to reach 4 METS are at increased risk and our work suggests that patients unable to meet a 3-MET demand at *AT* are at an increased risk. Most estimates of METS are based on treadmill exercise studies where METS are literally estimated not measured. The "Clinical Exercise Stress Testing—Safety and Performance Guidelines" published in the *Medical Journal of Australia* in 1996[17] suggest that METS may be estimated from nomograms. We would challenge this statement because such estimations are woefully inaccurate. Kleber et al.[18] have acknowledged that CPET is the "gold standard" for evaluation of cardiac failure, and the guidelines state that CPET has proved to be reliable and important in evaluation of patients with heart failure. Clearly if one is able to accurately measure $\dot{V}O_2$, then one has the "gold standard" for evaluation of cardiac failure. In fact the American College of Cardiology/American Heart Association guidelines for exercise testing state *"One of the strongest and most consistent prognostic markers identified in exercise testing is maximum exercise capacity, which is at least partly influenced by the extent of resting left ventricular function and the amount of further left ventricular dysfunction induced by exercise."*

Alternatives to CPET as a Screening Test

We recently published a review article in which we evaluate various preoperative screening tests.[19] Exercise electrocardiographic (ECG) testing

Table 1

Anaerobic Threshold (mL/kg/min) for 846 Patients*					
	Average	SD	Median	Range–Low	Range–High
Anaerobic Threshold	12.4	2.9	12.0	5.5	22
Peak V̇O$_2$	15.2	3.1			

*Average age 68, SD 9.9

is by far the most common test prescribed preoperatively. It can evaluate myocardial ischemia and estimate METS. One author suggests that a patient who achieves an estimated 7 METS or a heart rate >130 is low risk.[20] This equates to a V̇O$_2$ of 25 mL/kg/min. In our series of elderly patients, the measured average peak V̇O$_2$ for 846 patients was 15.2 mL/kg/min (Table 1). These differences occur because estimation of METS from treadmill grade or time is quite inaccurate, the METS being overestimated. This is particularly true in patients with heart disease, because of an increased reliance on anaerobic regeneration of high-energy phosphate (See chapter 1). A direct measure of V̇O$_2$ is required.

Ejection fraction determinations, by any means, do not correlate with aerobic capacity, with or without myocardial ischemia.[21,22] A low ejection fraction with an enlarged heart may well be associated with a normal stroke volume.

Transthoracic echocardiography is noninvasive and easy to perform, but the Perioperative Ischemia Research Group[23] failed to support the use of this technique in assessment of cardiac risk preoperatively. The same group found that dipyridamole-thallium scintigraphy was not a valid screening test for detection of postoperative cardiac events—even in vascular surgery patients.[24]

Dobutamine stress echocardiography has good sensitivity for detection of myocardial ischemia but does not allow for accurate assessment of functional capacity. The test is very expensive and interpretation is operator dependent.[20]

CPET has the advantage of being inexpensive, noninvasive, and applicable to most patients regardless of age. It is quick to perform and able to detect myocardial ischemia and evaluate cardiac and respiratory function objectively. There is no volitional component to the test, so the patient is not able to "cheat." Finally, the test is extremely repeatable and minimally open to subjective interpretation by the examiner.

Diagnosis of Myocardial Ischemia and Cardiac Failure by CPET

CPET involves the computerized analysis of gas exchange data during exercise. The computer is usually configured by the operator to perform many different analyses.

_____ Table 2 _____

Classification of Cardiac Failure by Cardiopulmonary Exercise Testing

Class	Definition	Peak $\dot{V}O_2$ (mL/kg/min)	AT (mL/kg/min)
A	No cardiac failure	>20	>14
B	Mild cardiac failure	16–19.9	11–13.9
C	Moderate cardiac failure	10–15.9	8–10.9
D	Severe cardiac failure	<10	<8

AT = anaerobic threshold. From reference 24.

Evaluation of cardiac function is usually performed by determination of the AT, the peak $\dot{V}O_2$, the $\dot{V}O_2$/heart rate (O_2 pulse) relationship, and the $\dot{V}O_2$/work rate relationship. Peak $\dot{V}O_2$ is not always the same as $\dot{V}O_2$max and many people fail to distinguish between the two. $\dot{V}O_2$max is defined as the point where, despite increases in work rate, there is no further increase in $\dot{V}O_2$. Peak $\dot{V}O_2$ is the highest $\dot{V}O_2$ reached during a specific test and may or may not be the same as $\dot{V}O_2$max. It is extremely rare for any of our patients to reach $\dot{V}O_2$max, and thus most exercise testing performed on the elderly would be best described as symptom-limited peak $\dot{V}O_2$. We define cardiac failure in terms of the O_2 uptake at AT, using the classes suggested by Weber and Janicki[25] (Table 2). Respiratory function is evaluated by such relationships as the $\dot{V}E$/$\dot{V}O_2$ and analysis of flow volume loops during exercise as well as at rest.

In our laboratory, the patient is always monitored via a computerized ECG monitor (Mortara ELI-100XR, Mortara Instruments, Milwaukee, WI). This machine gives an interference-free 12-lead display as well as tracking and storing ST segment depression and slope. This information is printed out at the end of each test. The x-axis of all printouts is time in minutes; thus, we are able to see at which point in the test ST segment depression occurred and to establish the extent of that depression in millimeters. The criterion used for diagnosis of myocardial ischemia was >1-mm ST segment depression, 60 ms after the J-point. This was determined by the Mortara ECG machine and was not subject to observer bias. In a previous study,[16] a cardiologist, blinded to both the cardiopulmonary exercise test and the Mortara report, had reported all ECGs, thus validating the computer-generated reporting.

Incidence and Significance of Myocardial Ischemia and Cardiac Failure

The incidence of ischemia, using the above criteria, has been remarkably constant at about 25% throughout our studies (52/214, 24.3%; 44/187, 23.5%).[13,16] In our latest study, 51 of 186 (27%) patients tested fulfilled the

_____ Table 3 _____

Mortality Rates Associated with Ischemia and AT, 1993

AT (mL/kg/min)	No	With Ischemia	CVS Deaths	% Mortality
<11	55	19	8	42
>11	132	25	1	4
Totals	187	44	9	(p<0.01)

AT = anaerobic threshold; CVS = cardiovascular system.

ECG criteria for myocardial ischemia. In contrast, angina was very uncommon, almost all ischemia being diagnosed by the exercise ECG criteria. Some patients developed a supraventricular tachycardia that gave rise to symptoms limiting the exercise test.

The average $\dot{V}O_2$ during exercise of 850 elderly, presurgery patients, at peak exercise was 15.2 mL/kg/min with an AT of 12.4 mL/kg/min. The average oxygen extraction ratio (OER) of elderly patients during exercise is 50%. Even following major abdominal surgery, $\dot{V}O_2$ rarely exceeds 7 mL/kg/min (250 mL/M^2); however OER is normally only 30% at rest. For these reasons a direct comparison of peak exercise $\dot{V}O_2$ and postsurgery $\dot{V}O_2$ is impossible. For any specified postsurgery $\dot{V}O_2$, however, the cardiac output would need to be a minimum of 2.5 times higher than for the same $\dot{V}O_2$ during exercise, while maintaining a normal resting OER. To place this in perspective, we published a study in 1989[26] in which 9 patients were exercised and also monitored by pulmonary artery catheter and metabolic gas exchange to measure cardiac output. This study showed that the average cardiac output increased from 4.6 L/min (SD±0.3) to 9.3 L/min (SD±0.6) after 4 minutes of work at 50 W. The $\dot{V}O_2$ index rose from 114 mL/min/M^2 (SD±5) to 515 mL/min/M^2 (SD±30).

In 1993, we pointed out that just the presence of myocardial ischemia did not correlate with postoperative mortality[13] (Table 3). This study showed that if ischemia was associated with an AT of <11 mL/kg/min, then mortality was 42%. If the AT was >11 mL/kg/min, then mortality was only 4%. In 1999, we showed that, of 9 cardiovascular deaths in 548 elderly surgical patients, only 3 had myocardial ischemia while 7 of these 9 had cardiac failure defined as an AT <11 mL/kg/min. No patient with an AT >11 mL/kg/min died, even if they had associated myocardial ischemia.[14]

Myocardial ischemia tends to limit ventricular function. If ischemia occurs early in exercise, it is deemed the cause of the cardiac failure. If, however, ventricular function is good and the ischemia occurs late in exercise, then it is viewed differently. Then the exercise is deemed to have caused the ischemia. In reality, the issue is the same; myocardial ischemia, at whatever work rate it occurs, will limit ventricular function. One could argue that the limiting factor in all exercise is cardiac failure—whether at 20 W for an elderly patient or the inability to run a marathon in less than

_____ Table 4 _____

Onset of Ischemia and *AT* in mL/kg/min in Two Series, 1996 and 2000

Total Patients	With Ischemia	Average *AT* with Early Ischemia	Average *AT* with Late Ischemia
214[15]	52	10.4 (n=21)	13.9 (n=31)
186*	51	10.9 (n=7)	13.3 (n=44)

*Unpublished date. *AT* = anaerobic threshold.

2 hours in an athlete. The difference is relative. The failure to transport adequate O_2 to regenerate the high-energy phosphate needed to support normal contraction of the myocardium during exercise conditions (myocardial ischemia) is merely one cause of cardiac failure, at whatever level of work the failure occurs. Clearly, if the surgery causes a rise in myocardial oxygen demand to the equivalent point in exercise where ischemia became apparent, that patient is more likely to develop myocardial ischemia than is the patient in whom ischemia occurred at a much higher work rate.

From the viewpoint of clinical relevance, myocardial ischemia during CPET may be divided into two main groups. The first group exhibits ischemia generally within 2 minutes of the onset of exercise. The second group does not show ischemia until levels of exercise approaching or exceeding the *AT*.[16] In those patients in whom the ischemia occurs early, the average *AT* is 10.4 mL/kg/min compared to those patients with late ischemia, in whom it is 13.9 mL/kg/min. Our most recent study showed a similar pattern (Table 4). Early ischemia is therefore associated with a low *AT* and a high grade of cardiac failure (classes C and D, as defined by Weber and Janicki[25]).

From examination of Table 3, it should be clear that the association of myocardial ischemia and an *AT* of <11 mL/kg/min has a high morbidity. The presence of myocardial ischemia, as a sole variable, did not influence mortality. These data were taken from a paper published in 1993,[13] before sufficient knowledge was available to create a patient selection bias. The implication of this is discussed later in this chapter.

Table 5 shows the significance of early compared to late myocardial ischemia in the incidence of postoperative events. These 51 patients with

_____ Table 5 _____

Cardiovascular Morbidity and Mortality for 51 Patients with Myocardial Ischemia

Ischemia	n	Mean *AT* mL/kg/min	Post-Op Ischemia	CVS Morbidity	CVS Deaths
Early	7	10.9	4	4	1
Late	44	13.3	10	0	0

AT = anaerobic threshold; CVS = cardiovascular system.

ischemia represented 27% of our series of 186. Of these, 4 patients had postoperative cardiovascular mortality/morbidity, 3 needing treatment of a significant tachyarrhythmia. One of these 3 suffered an acute myocardial infarction and survived. The fourth patient suffered an acute myocardial infarction and died.

If myocardial ischemia is the precipitating factor for postoperative morbidity or mortality, then one would expect this would occur predominantly in the group with ischemia, regardless of whether the patient had cardiac failure. If cardiac failure is the precipitating factor, then one would expect the morbidity and mortality to occur predominantly in the group with low AT cardiac failure, regardless of whether the patient had ischemia. Reference to Tables 3 and 5 shows that the mortality and morbidity occur in the group with cardiac failure, i.e., AT <11 mL/kg/min.

In our 1999 study of more than 700 patients,[14] only 1 patient died of a myocardial infarction. Of the 9 cardiac-related deaths in this study, only 2 patients had myocardial ischemia preoperatively as shown by CPET. Eight patients died from cardiac complications, and of these, 6 had an AT of <11 mL/kg/min. Certainly early ischemia and a low AT is the worst combination, but even then, the main cause of death is cardiac failure rather than an acute myocardial event.

It is our contention, supported by analysis of more than 2000 patients since 1990, that cardiac failure is the precipitating factor for postoperative morbidity and mortality. Myocardial ischemia occurring late in exercise with otherwise good ventricular function does not appear to be associated with increased morbidity or mortality. The explanation for this is that, following surgery, the myocardial oxygen demand in many patients may not reach levels associated with myocardial ischemia, even allowing for the increased myocardial work consequent to the postoperative rise in $\dot{V}O_2$.

Influence of Cardiopulmonary Exercise on Selection of Patients for Surgery

We published our first paper relating to cardiopulmonary exercise and surgical mortality in 1993.[13] At that time there was no selection process, either by us or by the surgeons, as the concept of using cardiopulmonary exercise was new; consequently, we sent the patients to surgery with knowledge of their cardiopulmonary exercise test result but without understanding the risk involved. Many patients with an AT well below 11 mL/kg/min as well as ischemia therefore underwent major surgery. The mortality of patients with a low AT and ischemia was very high (Table 3). At that time, we were unable to accurately assess the temporal relationship between ischemia and AT, as we were subsequently able to do following the introduction of the Mortara ECG machine in 1993.

_____ **Table 6** _____

ICU Bed Use and Mortality per 100 Patients Older than 65 for Elective Major Abdominal Surgery—1985 to 1999

	<1985	<1989	<1992	<1994	<1995	<1999	>1999
Admitted to ICU	40*	100†	45‡	45‡	36‡	29‡	22‡
Total bed days in ICU	600	430	260	225	152	78	66
Average length of stay in ICU	15	4.3	5.7	5.0	4.2	2.7	3.0
Nonsurgical, postoperative mortality	19§	6	7	4	2	0	0.5

*All emergency admissions; †all cases admitted electively preoperatively; ‡triaged on basis of cardiopulmonary exercise study; §cause of death not positively ascertained as study was retrospective (see text). ICU = intensive care unit.

By the time we published our prospective study in 1999,[14] the surgeons were beginning to be influenced by mortality figures and the cardiopulmonary exercise test result. In other words, a selection bias was evolving. Initially this was an occult process, but currently it has gained considerable momentum to the point where the cardiopulmonary exercise test is often performed before the definitive surgical procedure is scheduled. Surgeons are now influenced by the presence of an *AT* in single figures associated with early myocardial ischemia. These patients are now referred to cardiologists with a view to angiography and possible myocardial revascularization.

In our latest study (Table 5), it is apparent that only 7 patients out of 186 were operated on with a combination of an *AT* of <11 mL/kg/min and early myocardial ischemia. In 1993 (Table 4), 19 out of 187 were operated on with ischemia and an *AT* of <11 mL/kg/min.

These changes are almost certainly secondary to the process of selection by the surgeons, as we make no effort to influence the decision for surgery. In other words, patients who are tested and found to have early ischemia and a low *AT* are operated on only if there is no alternative.

A selection process would only be vindicated if mortality figures actually improve by its use. Current mortality from cardiovascular causes has consistently improved at our hospital since 1988 (Table 6).

Current Patient Triage System

To be of value, a comprehensive evaluation should assess the patient risk and include recommendations for patient care based on these findings.

Up to the completion of this, our latest study, we have used a triage system for patients following cardiopulmonary exercise as shown in Figure 2. The basis of this is that the high-risk patients, i.e., those with an *AT* of <11 mL/kg/min (with or without ischemia), were always admitted to the ICU and invasively monitored via a pulmonary artery catheter. Patients defined as having "surgery-specific risk," e.g., abdominal aortic aneurysms,

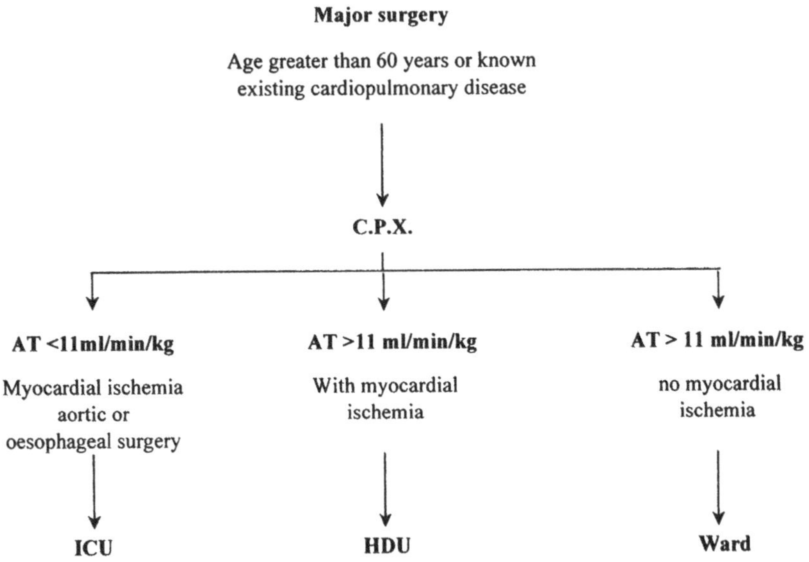

Major surgery

Age greater than 60 years or known
existing cardiopulmonary disease

↓

C.P.X.

AT <11ml/min/kg

Myocardial ischemia
aortic or
oesophageal surgery

↓

ICU

AT >11 ml/min/kg

With myocardial
ischemia

↓

HDU

AT > 11 ml/min/kg

no myocardial
ischemia

↓

Ward

Figure 2. Use of cardiopulmonary exercise (C.P.X.) testing for triage of elderly patients undergoing major surgery to the intensive care unit (ICU), high-dependency unit (HDU), and ward, based on anaerobic threshold (AT), evidence of myocardial ischemia, and type of surgery.

were also admitted to ICU. Those with an AT >11 mL/kg/min but with concomitant ischemia were admitted to a postsurgical high-dependency unit (HDU) for noninvasive monitoring.

Our latest study shows that patients in the latter group do not develop postsurgical cardiovascular complications. Consequently, we have now adopted a new triage system (Fig. 3), in which only patients with a low AT are admitted to ICU or HDU. Those patients with a low AT and myocardial ischemia are routinely referred to the cardiologists for assessment via angiography, where indicated. Patients with an AT >11 mL/kg/min are sent to the ward if they do not comply with the definition of surgery-specific risk.

Summary

The late 1970s and early 1980s saw an explosion in high technology in industry. This was not the case in the more conservative area of medicine. At that time, ICUs accepted many postsurgical patients, but only after they had deteriorated on the ward, often to the point of multisystem failure. Consequently, both mortality and morbidity were high. Through this period, many papers reported that postoperative mortality was extremely high in elderly patients with preexisting cardiac or pulmonary disease who were undergoing major surgery. Our own published studies supported this.

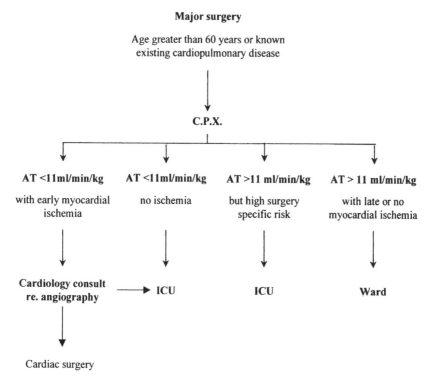

Figure 3. Current system for postoperative triage of elderly patients to ward or intensive care unit (ICU) based on anaerobic threshold (AT), early myocardial ischemia, and late or no myocardial ischemia.

Since 1988, we have used CPET as a preoperative screening test in the elderly to detect the presence of cardiac failure and/or myocardial ischemia. In a series of articles, we have shown that, as an independent variable, myocardial ischemia is not the major cause of perioperative mortality. By far, the most important issue is the presence of cardiac failure. We have also shown that tests such as ejection fraction, stress echocardiography, or transthoracic echocardiography are unreliable as screening tests. Age as a sole variable is also misleading and unreliable; cardiac function and age are not linear correlates.

Our latest study shows that the combination of cardiac failure, defined as an *AT* of <11 mL/kg/min, combined with early myocardial ischemia defines the patients at highest risk. The presence of myocardial ischemia in the absence of cardiac failure appears not to be a risk factor, whereas cardiac failure in the absence of myocardial ischemia does carry a higher risk of morbidity or mortality.

As a result of these findings, we set up a triage system whereby high-risk surgical patients and patients with *AT* <11 mL/kg/min are admitted to the ICU, and lower risk patients are sent to an HDU or the ward. Based on our most recent findings, we send patients with no evidence of cardiac failure (*AT* >11mL/kg/min) to the ward, even if they do exhibit myocardial ischemia at levels of exercise above this level.

During the 1990s, a process of selecting patients based on cardiopulmonary exercise evolved. This process has been occult, with the surgeons reluctant to operate on patients with an *AT* in single figures and concomitant myocardial ischemia, as this group of patients did not do well. In the same period, mortality dropped from 6% to 1%–2% or less.

Any system of preoperative evaluation should not only identify the presence of cardiac failure and/or myocardial ischemia, but should be capable of defining patient care based on these findings.

References

1. Knaus WA, Draper EA. APACHE II: a severity of disease classification system. Crit Care Med 1985;13:818-829.
2. Knaus WA, Draper EA. Prognosis in acute organ-system failure. Ann Surg 1985;6:685-693.
3. Clowes GHA, Del Guercio LRM. Circulatory response to trauma of surgical operations. Metabolism 1960;9:67-81.
4. Shoemaker WC. Cardiorespiratory patterns of surviving and non-surviving postoperative patients. Surg Gynecol Obstet 1972;134:810-814.
5. Goldman L, Caldera DL. Multifactorial index of cardiac risk in non-cardiac surgical procedures. N Engl J Med 1977;297:845-850.
6. Del Guercio LRM, Cohn JD. Monitoring operative risk in the elderly. JAMA 1980;243:1350-1355.
7. Older PO, Smith R. Experience with the preoperative invasive measurement of haemodynamic, respiratory and renal function in 100 elderly patients scheduled for major abdominal surgery. Anaesth Intensive Care 1988;16:389-395.
8. Buck N, Devlin HB, Lunn JN. The Report of a Confidential Enquiry into Perioperative Deaths. London: The Nuffield Provincial Hospitals Trust and the Kings Fund; 1987.
9. Wasserman K. Preoperative evaluation of cardiovascular reserve in the elderly. Chest 1993;104:663-664.
10. Poldermans D, Boersma E, Bax JJ. The effect of bisoprolol on perioperative mortality and myocardial infarction in high risk patients undergoing vascular surgery. Dutch Echocardiographic Cardiac Risk Evaluation Applying Stress Echocardiography Study Group. N Engl J Med 1999;341:1789-1794.
11. Mangano DT. Effect of atenolol on mortality and cardiovascular morbidity after non-cardiac surgery. Multicenter Study of Perioperative Ischemia Research Group. N Engl J Med 1996;335:1713-1720.
12. Beattie C, Fleisher LA. Perioperative myocardial ischemia and infarction. Int Anaesthesiol Clin 1992;30(1).
13. Older P, Smith R, Courtney P, Hone R. Preoperative evaluation of cardiac failure and ischemia in elderly patients by cardiopulmonary exercise testing. Chest 1993; 104:701-704.
14. Older P, Hall A, Hader R. Cardiopulmonary exercise testing as a screening test for perioperative management of major surgery in the elderly. Chest 1999; 116:355-362.

15. Eagle KA, Brunage BH, Chaitman BR, Ewy GA, Fleisher LA, Hertzer NR. Guidelines for perioperative cardiovascular evaluation for noncardiac surgery. Report of the American College of Cardiology/American Heart Association Task Force on Practice Guidelines. Committee on Perioperative Cardiovascular Evaluation for Noncardiac Surgery. Circulation 1996;93:1278-1317.

16. Older PO, Hall AC. The role of cardiopulmonary exercise testing for preoperative evaluation of the elderly. In: Wasserman K (ed): Exercise Gas Exchange in Heart Disease. Armonk, NY: Futura Publishing Co.; 1996:287-297.

17. Clinical exercise stress testing—safety and performance guidelines. The Cardiac Society of Australia and New Zealand. Med J Aust 1996;164:282-284.

18. Kleber FX, Sabin GV, Winter UJ, Reindl I, Beil S. Angiotensin-converting enzyme inhibitors in preventing remodeling and development of heart failure acute myocardial infarction: results of the German multicenter study of the effects of captopril on cardiopulmonary exercise parameters (ECCE). Am J Cardiol 1997;80:162A-167A.

19. Older P, Smith R, Hall A, French C. Preoperative cardiopulmonary risk assessment by cardiopulmonary exercise testing. Crit Care Resuscitation 2000;2:55-65.

20. Hollenberg SM. Preoperative cardiac risk assessment. Chest 1999;115:51S-57S.

21. Froelicher VF. Interpretation of specific exercise test responses. In: Froelicher VF (ed): Exercise and the Heart. 2nd ed. Chicago: Year Book Medical Publishers; 1987:83-145.

22. Dunselman PH, Kuntze CE, Van Bruggen A, Beekhuis H, Piers B, Scaf AH. Value of New York Heart Association classification, radionuclide ventriculography, and cardiopulmonary exercise tests for selection of patients for congestive heart failure studies. Am Heart J 1988;116:1475-1482.

23. Halm EA, Browner WS, Tubau JF, Tateo IM, Mangano DT. Echocardiography for assessing cardiac risk in patients having noncardiac surgery. Study of Perioperative Ischemia Research Group. Ann Intern Med 1996;125:433-441.

24. Mangano DT, Hollenberg M, Fegert G, Meyer ML, London MJ, Tubau JF. Perioperative myocardial ischemia in patients undergoing noncardiac surgery: incidence and severity during the 4 day perioperative period. The Study of Perioperative Ischemia (SPI) Research Group. J Am Coll Cardiol 1991;17:843-850.

25. Weber KT, Janicki JS. Cardiopulmonary exercise testing for evaluation of chronic cardiac failure. Am J Cardiol 1985;55:22A-31A.

26. McGrath BP, Newman R, Older P. Hemodynamic study of short- and long-term Isradapine treatment in patients with chronic ischemic congestive cardiac failure. Am J Med 1989;86(suppl 4A):75-80.

Section 3

Disease-Specific Abnormalities in Exercise Gas Exchange

10

Lung Diffusion Abnormalities and Exercise Capacity in Heart Failure

Pier Giuseppe Agostoni, MD, PhD
and Maurizio Bussotti, MD

Several recently published papers report a correlation between exercise capacity and lung diffusion abnormalities in heart failure patients.[1-4] Furthermore, in these patients, evidence suggests that behavior of gas diffusion across the alveolar-capillary membrane influences exercise capacity. Indeed, 1) clinical and exercise capacity improvement with some drugs, such as angiotensin-converting enzyme (ACE) inhibitors, correlates with the drug-induced increase in lung diffusion capacity for carbon monoxide (D_{LCO})[5]; 2) oxygen uptake ($\dot{V}_{O_2}$) kinetics can be altered with lung diffusion manipulation as done by binding carbon monoxide to hemoglobin and assessing the time constant of $\dot{V}_{O_2}$ in response to exercise[6]; and 3) exercise performance can be improved in heart failure patients by exercising patients below sea level, for example at the Dead Sea,[7] or with increased inspired oxygen fraction or with positive pressure ventilation.[8,9]

Unlike in patients with pulmonary diseases or intracardiac shunt or in elite athletes, however, exercise-induced hemoglobin desaturation is a rare event in patients with heart failure.[10,11] In reality, systemic artery partial pressure of O_2 (P_{O_2}) increases, as end-tidal P_{O_2} does, and hemoglobin saturation remains constant or slightly increases in heart failure patients at peak exercise.[12,13] Arterial O_2 content (CaO_2) also increases, mainly because of hemoconcentration, and can account for approximately 20% of the increase in arteriovenous O_2 content difference during exercise.[12,13] In other words, the value of oxygen delivery increment at peak exercise due to P_{O_2} increase is trivial, being on the flat upper part of the oxyhemoglobin dissociation

From Wasserman K (ed): *Cardiopulmonary Exercise Testing and Cardiovascular Health.*
Armonk, NY: Futura Publishing Company, Inc.; © 2002.

_____ Table 1 _____

Exercise-Induced Increase in Hemoglobin and Plasma Proteins at Peak Exercise in Normal Subjects and Patients with Heart Failure

Variable	Normal Subjects	Heart Failure Patients
Number of subjects	50	50
Peak oxygen consumption (mL/kg/min)	33±7	16±4*
Hemoglobin increase (g/dL)	1.1±0.5	0.6±0.4*
Hematocrit increase (%)	3±1	2±1*
Lactate increase (mmol/L)	8.3±4.2	4.3±2.2*
Plasma protein increase (g/dL)	0.8±0.3	0.4±0.3*

*$p<0.01$ from normal subjects. Data from reference 14.

curve. The exercise-induced increase in hemoglobin is seen in heart failure patients and normal subjects and occurs above the anaerobic threshold.[14-16] An increment in hematocrit can result from fluid flow from the intravascular to the extra vascular space and/or to recruitment of red blood cells from the spleen.[17-19] In a recent report,[14] we observed that the increase in red blood cells was paralleled by an increase in plasma proteins suggesting fluid movement from the vascular space is probably the major cause of the exercise-induced increase in red blood cell (Table 1). The driving force is likely an increase in intracellular osmotic forces due to lactate or lactate metabolite increases. Accordingly, since normal subjects have a greater muscle mass and, if compared to patients with severe heart failure, a greater lactic acid plasma level at peak exercise, which reflects a greater intracellular lactic acid level, the increase in red blood cell per 100 mL of blood is greater in normal subjects compared to heart failure patients (Table 1). It is still possible that recruitment of red blood cells from the spleen plays a minor role in the increase in red blood cell count per unit of blood in humans.[19]

Exercise Capacity and Diffusion Capacity in Heart Failure

The physiological link between exercise capacity and DLCO in heart failure patients leaves uncertain a cause/effect relationship. Consequently, little care has been dedicated to the understanding of the clinical meaning of lung diffusion abnormalities in heart failure patients.

A major problem lies in the fact that lung diffusion capacity has been considered a fixed entity for a given individual. However, this concept is not true. Indeed, some drugs, such as ACE inhibitors and cyclosporine, actively interfere with the DLCO, which increases with the former[5] and decreases with the latter.[20] On the other hand, exercise also changes DLCO.[4] In fact, all of the variables that affect DLCO undergo changes with exercise. Consequently, DLCO varies during exercise. In reality:

$$1/\text{DLCO} = 1/\text{Dm} + 1/\vartheta\text{Vc}$$

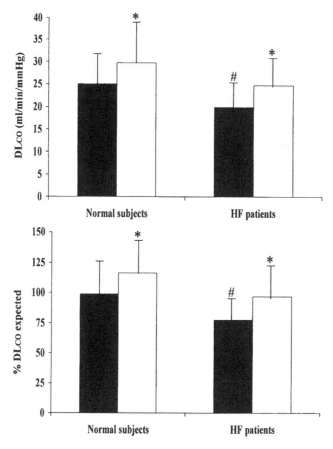

Figure 1. Lung diffusing capacity for carbon monoxide (DLCO) at rest (black columns) and during constant workload exercise (5 minutes, empty columns) as absolute value (upper panel) or as a percentage of predicted normal resting DLCO value (lower panel). Exercise data were obtained at a workload equal to 20% of peak O_2 consumption. Data are mean ± SD of 20 normal subjects (left) and 20 heart failure (HF) subjects (right) in stable clinical conditions.

where DLCO is the total pulmonary diffusion to carbon monoxide, Dm is membrane diffusion, and ϑVc is red cell diffusion with ϑ being the rate of carbon monoxide uptake by the red cells and Vc the pulmonary capillary blood volume. It is not easy to measure DLCO during exercise. Presently, reliable measurements can only be obtained during constant workload exercise with exercise performed at low workload. Therefore, only very limited qualitative and no quantitative analysis of exercise-induced DLCO changes has been done. We know that at 20% of peak $\dot{V}O_2$, DLCO increases in both normal subjects and patients with moderate to severe heart failure (Fig. 1), with the resting DLCO value being lower in heart failure patients. However, our knowledge of the DLCO behavior during exercise is limited; indeed, we do not know: 1) whether the increase of D_{LCO} observed with a workload equal to 20% of peak O_2 consumption is the maximal possible exercise-induced D_{LCO} increase; 2) whether the D_{LCO} increase is progressive with workload increase; 3) whether D_{LCO} during exercise has a different behavior in patients versus normal subjects; and 4) whether at peak exercise, D_{LCO} actually increases or decreases.

Technically, molecular diffusion for carbon monoxide across the alveolar-capillary membrane and pulmonary capillary blood volume can be measured according to the Roughton and Forster method.[21] For this purpose a gas mixture with 0.3% methane, 0.3% carbon monoxide, and 0.3% acetylene balanced with nitrogen with 3 different O_2 concentrations equal to 20%, 40%, and 60%, respectively, are usually used. After a deep breath, subjects are asked to perform a constant low expiratory flow maneuver; to facilitate this, a small expiratory flow resistance is usually applied. A different technique has been used by Smith et al.,[4] but again during constant low workload exercise. These investigators used a rebreathing technique with a gas mixture containing 35% O_2, 3% sulfur hexafluoride, 0.3% acetylene, and 0.3% carbon monoxide, with the balance being nitrogen. This technique requires a lot of expertise and some nonphysiological conditions (the tidal breathing must be 10% to 15% higher than needed) and allows measurements of D_{LCO} and effective pulmonary blood flow.

Mechanism of D_{LCO} Changes

Exercise-induced increase in D_{LCO} can be due to increase in capillary volume through recruitment of new vessels, increase in red blood cells per unit of lung capillary blood volume, and increase in Dm. The latter is observed mainly in heart failure patients who, at 20% of peak $\dot{V}O_2$, increase the molecular diffusion for carbon monoxide across the alveolar-capillary membrane by ~25%, which has statistical relevance. Normal subjects show a tendency to increase by only ~10%. This difference remains the same even if molecular diffusion for carbon monoxide is normalized for alveolar volume. The cause of this difference is not known; several hypotheses can be proposed including an increased shear stress effect on the alveolar-capillary membrane, an increase in nitric oxide, and prostacyclin release due to exercise-induced changes in thoracic movements, pressure, capillary volume, or blood flow. We have, intentionally, not quoted possible exercise-induced changes in ϑ because no data are available on this variable; however, changes in ϑ resulting from Bohr effect for work rates below anaerobic threshold, where the D_{LCO} measurements were done, are unlikely. But besides the shape of the oxyhemoglobin dissociation curve, other factors can influence ϑ, including red blood cell shape and thickness of red blood cells on alveolar-capillary membrane.

___ **Table 2** ___

Effects of Posture on Lung Diffusion in 12 Patients with Chronic Heart Failure

Posture	D_{LCO}	VA	D_{LCO}/VA	Dm	Vc
Sitting	23 ± 2*	5.3 ± 1.7*	4.4 ± 1.4	34 ± 2	107 ± 28
Prone	23 ± 3	5.2 ± 1.4	4.4 ± 0.3	32 ± 1	137 ± 70
Supine	22 ± 1	5.0 ± 1.2	4.4 ± 1.1	31 ± 4	115 ± 19

*$p < 0.05$ versus supine. D_{LCO} = lung diffusion for carbon monoxide (mL/min/mm Hg); Dm = alveolar capillary membrane diffusive properties (mL/min/mm Hg); VA = alveolar volume (L); Vc = lung capillary blood volume (mL).

Lung diffusion and lung mechanical characteristics are usually related to each other at rest and during exercise. Several papers[22-24] have reported resting evaluations of D_{LCO} and of standard pulmonary function tests, but data on relationship between the two during effort are almost lacking. In patients with moderate heart failure, resting D_{LCO} is slightly reduced due to a reduction in Dm with a normal Vc. If heart failure is severe, reduction in Dm is greater and only partially compensated by an increase in Vc.[2]

Several variables influence D_{LCO}. First, D_{LCO} decreases with age[25] because of a reduction in both Vc and Dm. Second, body position influences D_{LCO}, which increases because of an increase in Vc.[26] This is true in normal subjects but not in patients with heart failure (Table 2). Beside the effect of body position on blood volume in the lung it is also likely that 1) the weight of a heavy heart above or below a significant proportion of the lungs plays a role in determining D_{LCO} by reducing lung volume available for gas exchange; and 2) the volume occupied by an enlarged heart influences lung volumes as well as lung mechanical and diffusive properties. Indeed, there is a strong negative correlation between D_{LCO} and the cardiothoracic index, a value that correlates the heart to chest size.[27] Similarly, there is a strong negative correlation between each of alveolar volume, vital capacity, forced expiratory volume in 1 second, and the cardiothoracic index.[27]

On the other hand, pulmonary function tests have been performed immediately post exercise. In normal subjects but not in heart failure patients, pulmonary function improves post exercise, likely due to bronchodilatation. Possible causes are exercise-induced increase in catecholamines and a stretch effect on the bronchi and lung resistive units induced by the exercise increase in ventilation. An example is reported in Figure 2. The left panel shows the flow/volume curve of two maximal inspiratory/expiratory maneuvers obtained from a patient with heart failure. The two curves were obtained before and immediately after an exercise test. The two curves are superimposable. In the right panel, the same maneuvers have been repeated in a normal subject; in this case, the flow/volume curve is larger after exercise. This explains why the flow/volume loop recorded at peak exercise in normal

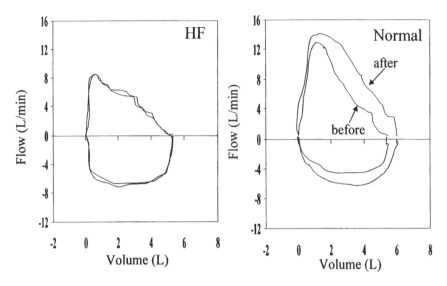

Figure 2. Flow/volume curve of two maximal inspiratory/expiratory maneuvers obtained before and immediately after a maximal exercise. In the left panel, measurements were obtained from a patient with heart failure. In the right panel, the same measurements were obtained in a normal subject. The two curves are the same in the heart failure patient, but flow/volume loop is larger after exercise in the normal subject.

subjects and particularly athletes can show a loop that exceeds the one measured during the maximal inspiratory/expiratory maneuver at rest.[11]

Effect of Treatment of Heart Failure on DLCO

Therapy can differently influence DLCO and standard pulmonary function. A first example can be obtained by comparing angiotensin-receptor (AT$_1$) blockers and ACE inhibitors. In the early clinical studies AT$_1$ blockers have been suggested as an alternative treatment for patients who cannot be treated with ACE inhibitors; an example is ACE-inhibitor-related cough.[28] Although "inhibitors" and "blockers" both improve exercise performance, pulmonary function at rest and DLCO are positively influenced only by the ACE inhibitor. Similarly, pulmonary function during exercise (ratio of dead space to tidal volume) seems to improve to a greater extent with ACE inhibitors.[29] Furthermore, ACE inhibitors and AT$_1$ blockers are now used together in heart failure treatment.[30] The action of ACE inhibitors on diffusive lung function is related to the fact that ACE inhibitors act on both ACE and kinase II, an enzyme which is highly concentrated in the lungs, particularly on the luminal surface of the pulmonary vasculature.[31]

A second example of how therapy can differently influence DLCO and standard pulmonary function is heart transplant. Heart transplant is probably the most effective treatment for advanced heart failure. Usually 1 year after successful surgery, patients significantly improve in terms of standard pulmonary function at rest and exercise capacity.[32-35] Strangely enough, improvement in exercise capacity and lung mechanics, both at rest and during exercise, is not accompanied by an improvement in lung diffusion. Actually, shortly after heart transplant, D_{LCO} is reduced compared to presurgery values. The negative effect of cyclosporine treatment on D_{LCO} has been considered responsible for the reduced D_{LCO}. Recently Mettauer et al.[35] suggested that both severity and duration of heart failure may interfere with diffusing capacity and that, in chronic heart failure, the alveolar-capillary membrane might undergo irreversible changes.

Figure 3. Diagram of the ultrafiltration circuit used to remove body fluid. The technique acts via a filter allocated in a veno-venous bypass circuit where blood is propelled by a peristaltic pump; the filter allows separation of blood and plasma water which contains substances with a molecular weight lower than 50.000 d.

To better understand this problem, we recently performed a study aimed at evaluating the effects of ultrafiltration on D_{LCO}.[36] Indeed, ultrafiltration is a technique that allows reduction in fluid content of the body, and particularly lung fluid content, in patients with heart failure. This technique acts via a filter allocated in a veno-venous bypass circuit where blood is propelled by a peristaltic pump; the filter allows separation of blood and plasma water that contains substances with a molecular weight lower than 50.000 d (Fig. 3).[37] Ultrafiltration is done without any fluid replacement. Neither diuretics nor ultrafiltration are able to improve D_{LCO}, but ultrafiltration improves forced vital capacity, forced expiratory volume in 1 second, and maximal voluntary ventilation in patients with chronic heart failure.[37-39] Figures 4 and 5 report the data from ultrafiltration. Pre-ultrafiltration data in patients with severe heart failure show a significant reduction in vital capacity, maximal voluntary ventilation, forced expiratory volume, D_{LCO}, and specific Dm, and an increase in lung tissue volume (measured from constant expiratory flow decay curves of carbon monoxide, acetylene, and methane) and capillary blood volume. As a whole, these data suggest the presence of a restrictive disease.[40] Four days after a successful procedure, resting pulmonary function, reflecting lung mechanics, improves. Lung tissue volume is decreased, obviously reflecting a decrease in lung water content; however, D_{LCO} and its subcomponents remain unchanged (Fig. 5). This observation suggests that the alveolar-capillary membrane undergoes changes unrelated to the alveolar-capillary membrane water content, but more likely related to cellular and connective content in chronic heart failure.[35]

Besides the effects of ACE inhibitors, other factors affect the diffusive characteristics of the alveolar-capillary membrane in patients with chronic congestive heart failure. Infusion of even a small amount of saline (150 mL) induces a transient reduction of D_{LCO} in patients but not in normal subjects

_____ Table 3 _____

Effects of Saline Infusion on D_{LCO}, Dm, and Vc in Normal Subjects and Heart Failure Patients

	Pre-Infusion	150 mL Saline	750 mL Saline
Normal subjects			
D_{LCO}	34.5±0.6	34.3±0.6	34.6±0.5
Dm	49±2	50±3	50±3
Vc	146±25	145±20	143±22
Heart failure patients			
D_{LCO}	23.1±1.0*	22.1±0.0*†	21.2±1.2*†
Dm	30±1*	28±2*†	28±3*†
Vc	141±31	158±28†	161±38†

D_{LCO} = lung diffusing capacity for carbon monoxide (mL/min/mm Hg); Dm = membrane diffusing capacity (mL/min/mm Hg); Vc = capillary volume (mL). *p<0.01 from normal subjects; †p<0.01 from pre-infusion. Data from reference 41.

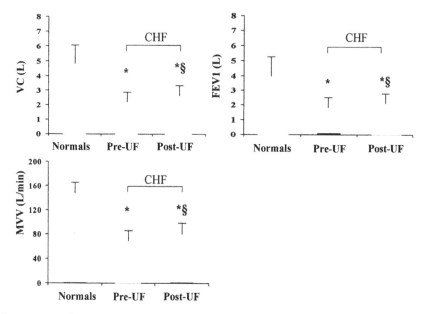

Figure 4. Vital capacity (VC), maximal voluntary ventilation (MVV), and forced expiratory volume in 1 second (FEV1) in normal subjects and in heart failure patients (CHF) before and 4 days after ultrafiltration (UF). *p<0.01 from normal subjects, §p<0.01 from pre-ultrafiltration.

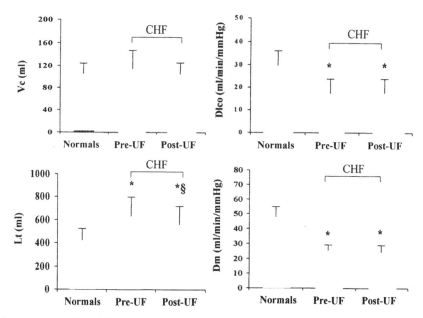

Figure 5. Capillary blood volume (Vc), lung diffusing capacity for carbon monoxide (Dlco), lung tissue volume (Lt), and specific membrane diffusion for carbon monoxide (Dm) in normal subjects and in heart failure patients (CHF) before and 4 days after ultrafiltration (UF). *p<0.01 from normal subjects, §p<0.01 from pre-ultrafiltration.

_____ **Table 4** _____

Effects of Glucose Infusion on D_{LCO}, Dm, and Vc in Heart Failure Patients

	Pre-Infusion	150 mL Glucose	750 mL Glucose
D_{LCO}	23.0±0.9	23.8±0.6	23.5±0.8
Dm	28±1	30±2	33±3*
Vc	142±24	129±25	125±28

D_{LCO} = lung diffusing capacity for carbon monoxide (mL/min/mm Hg); Dm = membrane diffusing capacity (mL/min/mm Hg); Vc = capillary volume (mL). *p<0.05 from pre-infusion. Data from reference 41.

(Table 3). An infusion of a greater amount of saline has similar effects. It is, at first glance, surprising that if solute infused is glucose instead of NaCl, D_{LCO} remains constant (Table 4). The increase in Dm with glucose infusion, however, suggests an improvement of membrane conductance and speaks in favor of an active co-transport of water and solutes across the alveolar-capillary membrane.[41]

Effects of Altitude on D_{LCO}

D_{LCO} may severely influence exercise capacity at altitude. As altitude increases, the inspiratory PO_2 decreases. The acute effects of altitude on exercise capacity can be studied in laboratories at high altitude [42,43] but also easily mimicked in those at sea level.[44] It is of clinical relevance to inform normal subjects and patients about the amount of exercise capacity reduction they might expect at a given altitude.[45] Hypoxia studies can also provide an understanding of the physiology underlying the interrelation between D_{LCO} and exercise capacity. Indeed, because the oxyhemoglobin dissociation curve is overall S shaped, but linearly-shaped between a PO_2 of 40 and 80 mm Hg, in hypoxia the correlation between PO_2 and oxyhemoglobin saturation with D_{LCO} is easier to study and understand. Furthermore, hypoxia should magnify the role of diffusion impairment on exercise capacity. Accordingly, we studied the correlations, both at rest and during exercise, among D_{LCO}, O_2 delivery, and exercise capacity during normoxic and hypoxic conditions in heart failure patients and in normal subjects.[45] O_2 delivery depends on cardiac output, systemic artery PO_2, hemoglobin concentration, and shape of oxyhemoglobin dissociation curve. All of these factors undergo exercise-induced changes. D_{LCO} reflects lung gas exchange surface area and alveolar-arterial O_2 pressure difference [$\Delta P(A-aO_2)$].

As already reported, resting D_{LCO} and peak $\dot{V}O_2$ correlated in normoxic conditions (inspired O_2 fraction = 0.21) in heart failure patients (n=40) but not in normal subjects (n=40). With hypoxia (we used an inspired O_2 fraction = 0.16 mimicking an altitude of ~2000 m/~6000′), this correlation further increased in patients (i.e., resting D_{LCO} correlated to peak $\dot{V}O_2$ obtained in

_____ Table 5 _____

Correlations between CaO_2 and D_{LCO} and between CaO_2 and peak $\dot{V}O_2$ in 20 Heart Failure Patients

	CaO_2 vs. D_{LCO}	CaO_2 vs. Peak $\dot{V}O_2$
Heart failure patients		
Normoxia	R=0.499	R=0.557
Peak exercise	p<0.03	p<0.01
Hypoxia	R=0.500	R=0.542
Peak exercise	p<0.03	p<0.01
Normal subjects		
Normoxia	R=0.405	R=0.391
Peak exercise	p=NS	p=NS
Hypoxia	R=0.481	R=0.430
Peak exercise	p<0.03	p=0.06

D_{LCO} = lung diffusing capacity for carbon monoxide; CaO_2 = arterial oxygen content; NS = not significant.

hypoxic condition). It is noteworthy that D_{LCO} also correlated with exercise capacity during hypoxia in normal subjects (Table 5). In the same tests, arterial O_2 content correlated with resting D_{LCO} and peak $\dot{V}O_2$ in patients with normoxia and with hypoxia, and in normal subjects only with hypoxia (Table 5). Table 6 shows PO_2, oxyhemoglobin saturation, O_2 content, and alveolar-arterial O_2 pressure difference. With hypoxia, further oxyhemoglobin desaturation occurs during exercise in normal subjects and in patients.

_____ Table 6 _____

Hemoglobin Concentration, PaO_2, Hb sat, CaO_2, and $P_{(A-aO_2)}$ at Rest and Peak Exercise in Normoxic and Hypoxic Conditions in Heart Failure Patients and Normal Subjects

	Normoxia: Rest	Normoxia: P. Exer.	Hypoxia: Rest	Hypoxia: P. Exer.
Heart failure patients				
PaO_2 (mm Hg)	86±6	99±11*	68±9†	61±8*†
Hb/O_2 sat (%)	97.2±0.8	97.7±1.2	94.9±2.0†	92.1±3.1*†
CaO_2	18.3±2.0	19.5±2.2*	18.1±1.9	18.5±2.3*†
$P_{(A-aO_2)}$	14.7±7.6	20.5±10.0*	11.1±8.8†	23.0±7.8*
Normal subjects				
PaO_2	92.3±6.0	98.4±8.3*	73.8±9.5†	66.8±7.6*†
Hb/O_2 sat	97.8±0.3	97.7±0.6	96.1±1.6†	93.7±2.2*†
CaO_2	18.1±1.5	19.3±1.3*	17.8±1.5†	18.7±1.4*†
$P_{(A-aO_2)}$	6.4±8.5	19.4±6.2*	4.5±6.6	21.5±5.7*

*p<0.05 versus rest, †p<0.05 versus normoxia. PaO_2 = arterial oxygen pressure; Hb/O_2 sat = hemoglobin saturation; CaO_2 = arterial oxygen content; $P_{(A-aO_2)}$ = alveolar-arterial pressure difference for oxygen.

The observed reduction of PO_2 and oxyhemoglobin saturation is counterbalanced by an increase in hemoglobin.[13]

Summary

In conclusion, although none of the present evidence considered separately proves a causal role of DLco impairment in generating the reduced exercise capacity of heart failure patients, the pathophysiology contributing to the reduction in DLco appears to also contribute to the reduced exercise capacity in heart failure patients.

References

1. Puri S, Baker BL, Oakley CM, Hughes JMB, Cleland JGF. Increased alveolar/capillary membrane resistance to gas transfer in patients with chronic heart failure. Br Heart J 1994;72:140-144.

2. Puri S, Baker BL, Dutka DP, Oakley CM, Hughes JM, Cleland JG. Reduced alveolar-capillary membrane diffusing capacity in chronic heart failure. Circulation 1995;91:2769-2774.

3. Guazzi M. Alveolar capillary membrane dysfunction in chronic heart failure: pathophysiology and therapeutic implication. Clin Sci 2000;98:633-641.

4. Smith AA, Cowburn PJ, Parker ME, et al. Impaired pulmonary diffusion during exercise in patients with chronic heart failure. Circulation 1999;100:1406-1410.

5. Guazzi M, Marenzi GC, Alimento M, Contini M, Agostoni PG. Improvement of alveolar capillary diffusing capacity in chronic heart failure and counteracting effects of aspirin. Circulation 1997;95:1930-1936.

6. Koike A, Wasserman K, McKenzie DK, Zanconato S, Weiler-Ravell D. Evidence that diffusion limitation determines oxygen uptake kinetics during exercise in humans. J Clin Invest 1990;86:1698-1706.

7. Abinader EG, Sharif DS, Goldhammer E. Effects of low altitude on exercise performance in patients with congestive heart failure after healing of acute myocardial infarction. Am J Cardiol 1999;83:383-387.

8. Moore DP, Weston AR, Hughes JMB, Oakley CM, Cleland JGF. Effects of increased inspired oxygen concentration on exercise performance in chronic heart failure. Lancet 1992;339:850-853.

9. O'Donnel DE, D'Arsigny C, Ray S, Abdollah H, Webb KA. Ventilatory assistance improves exercise endurance in stable congestive heart failure. Am J Respir Crit Care Med 1999;160:1804-1811.

10. Wagner PD. A theoretical analysis of factors determining $\dot{V}O_2MAX$ at sea level and altitude. Respir Physiol 1996;106:329-343.

11. Dempsey JA. Normal exercise physiology. In: Gallacher CG, Marciniuk DD (eds): Interpretation of Clinical Exercise Testing for the Clinician. American Thoracic Society 1997:1-19.

12. Agostoni PG, Wasserman K, Perego GB, et al. Oxygen transport to muscle during exercise in chronic congestive heart failure secondary to idiopathic dilated cardiomyopathy. Am J Cardiol 1997;79:1120-1124.

13. Perego GB, Marenzi GC, Guazzi M, et al. Contribution of PO_2, P50, and Hb to changes in arteriovenous O_2 content during exercise in heart failure. J Appl Physiol 1996;80:623-631.

14. Agostoni PG, Wasserman K, Guazzi M, et al. Exercise-induced hemoconcentration in heart failure due to dilated cardiomyopathy. Am J Cardiol 1999;83:278-280.

15. Stringer W, Wasserman K, Casaburi R, et al. Lactic acidosis as a facilitator of oxyhemoglobin dissociation during exercise. J Appl Physiol 1994;76:1462-1467.

16. Novosadova J. The changes in hematocrit, hemoglobin, plasma volume and proteins during and after different types of exercise. Eur J Appl Physiol Occup Physiol 1977;36:223-230.

17. Senay LC Jr, Rogers G, Jooste P. Changes in blood plasma during progressively treadmill and cycle exercise. J Appl Physiol 1980;49:59-65.

18. Jung T, Korotzer B, Stringer W, Jones A, Wasserman K. Lactate concentration increase and transcellular fluid flux during exercise. Am J Respir Crit Care Med 1996;153:A647.

19. Otto AC, Rona du Toit DJ, Pretorius H, Lötter MG, Van Aswegen A. The effect of exercise on normal splenic volume measured with SPECT. Clin Nucl Med 1995;20:884-887.

20. Casan P, Sanchis J, Cladellas M, Amergual MJ, Caralps JM. Diffusing lung capacity and cyclosporine. Ann Rev Med 1986;37:215-224.

21. Roughton FJW, Forster RE. Relative importance of diffusion and chemical reaction rates in determining rate of exchange of gases in the human lung, with special reference to true diffusing capacity of pulmonary membrane and volume of blood in the lung capillaries. J Appl Physiol 1957;11:290-302.

22. Light RW, George RB. Serial pulmonary function in patients with acute heart failure. Arch Intern Med 1983;143:429-433.

23. Chua TP, Coats AJS. The lungs in chronic heart failure. Eur Heart J 1995; 16:882-887.

24. Hosenpud JD, Stibolt TA, Atwal K, Shelley D. Abnormal pulmonary function specifically related to congestive heart failure: comparison of patients before and after cardiac transplantation. Am J Med 1990;88:493-496.

25. Lentner C. Geigy Scientific Tables. Vol. 3. Basel: Ciba-Geigy Limited; 1984:71-77.

26. Chang SC, Chang HI, Liu SY, Shiao GM, Perng RP. Effects of body position and age on membrane diffusing capacity and pulmonary capillary blood volume. Chest 1992;102:139-142.

27. Agostoni PG, Cattadori G, Guazzi M, Palermo P, Bussotti M, Marenzi G. Cardiomegaly as a possible cause of lung dysfunction in patients with heart failure. Am Heart J 2000;140:E24.

28. Pitt B. Effects of angiotensin II antagonists in comparison to ACE inhibitors in patients with heart failure due to systolic left ventricular dysfunction. Heart Fail Rev 1999;3:221-232.

29. Guazzi M, Melzi G, Agostoni PG. Comparison of change in respiratory function and exercise oxygen uptake with losartan vs. enalapril in congestive heart failure secondary to ischemic or idiopathic cardiomyopathy. Am J Cardiol 1997; 80:1572-1576.

30. Guazzi M, Palermo P, Pontone G, Susini F, Agostoni PG. Synergistic efficacy of enalapril and losartan on exercise performance and oxygen consumption at peak exercise in congestive heart failure. Am J Cardiol 1999;84:1038-1043.

31. Guazzi M, Marenzi GC, Melzi G, Agostoni P. Angiotensin-converting enzyme inhibition facilitates alveolar-capillary gas transfer and improves ventilation per-

fusion coupling in patients with left ventricular dysfunction. Clin Pharmacol Ther 1999;65:319-327.

32. Wright RS, Levine MS, Bellamy PE, et al. Ventilatory and diffusion abnormalities in potential heart transplant recipients. Chest 1990;98:816-820.

33. Naum CC, Sciurba FC, Rogers RM. Pulmonary function abnormalities in chronic severe cardiomyopathy preceding cardiac transplantation. Am Rev Respir Dis 1992;145:1334-1338.

34. Ravenscraft SA, Gross CR, Kubo SH, et al. Pulmonary function after successful heart transplantation. One year follow-up. Chest 1993;103:54-58.

35. Mettauer B, Lampert E, Charloux A, et al. Lung membrane diffusing capacity, heart failure, and heart transplantation. Am J Cardiol 1999;83:62-67.

36. Agostoni PG, Guazzi M, Bussotti M, Grazi M, Palermo P, Marenzi G. Lack of improvement of lung diffusing capacity following fluid withdrawal by ultrafiltration in chronic heart failure. J Am Coll Cardiol 2000;36:1600-1604.

37. Agostoni PG, Marenzi GC, Sganzerla P, et al. Lung-heart interaction as a substrate for the improvement in exercise capacity after body fluid volume depletion in moderate congestive heart failure. Am J Cardiol 1995;76:793-798.

38. Agostoni PG, Marenzi GC, Pepi M, et al. Isolated ultrafiltration in moderate congestive heart failure. J Am Coll Cardiol 1993;21:424-431.

39. Agostoni PG, Marenzi GC, Lauri G, et al. Sustained improvement in functional capacity after removal of body fluid with isolated ultrafiltration in chronic cardiac insufficiency: failure of furosemide to provide the same result. Am J Med 1994;96:191-199.

40. Wasserman K, Zhang YY, Gitt A, et al. Lung function and exercise gas exchange in chronic heart failure. Circulation 1997;96:2221-2227.

41. Guazzi M, Agostoni PG, Bussotti M, Guazzi MD. Impeded alveolar-capillary gas transfer with saline infusion in heart failure. Hypertension 1999;34:1202-1207.

42. Peacock AJ. Oxygen at high altitude. Br Med J 1998;317:1063-1066.

43. Gong HJ. Oxygen at altitude and on aircraft. In: Tiep BL (ed): Portable Oxygen Therapy: Including Oxygen Conserving Methodology. Mount Kisco, NY: Futura Publishing Co.; 1991:437-469.

44. Gong H, Tashkin DP, Lee EY, Simmons MS. Hypoxia-altitude simulation test. Evaluation of patients with chronic airway obstruction. Am Rev Respir Dis 1984;130:980-986.

45. Agostoni P, Cattadori G, Guazzi M, et al. Effects of simulated altitude-induced hypoxia on exercise capacity in patients with chronic heart failure. Am J Med 2000;109:450-455.

11

Cardiopulmonary and Metabolic Responses to Exercise in Patients with Hypertrophic Cardiomyopathy

Brian J. Whipp, PhD, DSc, Soraya Jones, PhD,
Perry M. Elliott, MD, Sanjay Sharma, MD,
and William J. McKenna, MD, DSc

Hypertrophic cardiomyopathy (HCM) is a heterogeneous disease characterized by increased left ventricular mass without demonstrable cause, and microscopic evidence of myofibrillar and myocyte disarray.[1,2] Although most patients remain asymptomatic, the most commonly reported symptoms are dyspnea, chest pain, palpitations, dizziness, and syncope. The most severe complication of HCM, however, is sudden death, with annual rates of 1% to 2% in the adult population and 2% to 4% in childhood and adolescence.[3-5]

Patients with HCM typically manifest exercise intolerance,[6,7] and laboratory studies have demonstrated low peak oxygen uptake (peak $\dot{V}O_2$) and lactate threshold (θ_L).[8,9] These characteristics, however, are also manifest in patients with a wide range of functional abnormalities associated with other cardiac, peripheral vascular, pulmonary, and various metabolic diseases, and even in normal but chronically sedentary people.[10,11] Such characteristics are consequently not discriminatory. In contrast, the profile of cardiopulmonary and metabolic responses to small-step incremental or ramp exercise test[12] that spans the tolerable work rate range at an optimized rate[13] may provide more subtle, and often discriminatory, evidence of abnormal physio-

From Wasserman K (ed): *Cardiopulmonary Exercise Testing and Cardiovascular Health.*
Armonk, NY: Futura Publishing Company, Inc.; © 2002.

logical functioning that is pathognomonic of particular systemic sources of exercise intolerance (for further discussion see references 10, 11, and 14).

Recently, with use of both age- and sex-matched control groups and normal predicted values from the literature as frames of reference, the normalcy, or otherwise, of such response profiles has been established in patients with HCM.[15,16]

Two large-cohort studies of the cardiopulmonary and metabolic responses to incremental ramp exercise in patients with HCM (aged between 12 and 62 years) have recently been reported by our group: 50 patients with HCM and 22 sedentary age- and sex-matched controls,[15] and 135 patients with HCM and 50 age- and sex-matched controls.[16] In both studies the diagnosis was based on conventional World Health Organization definitions[17] for probands and recently proposed criteria for first-degree relatives and obligate or proven gene carriers (approximately 20%).[18,19] In each case the groups consisted of consecutive patients who attended the cardiomyopathy clinic at our institution, who were in sinus rhythm with a normal blood pressure response to exercise, and who had not undergone myotomy-myectomy or pacemaker implantation. The patients were instructed not to take their cardiac-related medications (calcium channel blockers, beta-blockers, and disopyramide) for at least 48 hours prior to the exercise test; this was not the case for those taking amiodarone (7% and 14% of the patients of Jones et al.[15] and Sharma et al.[16], respectively) owing to its long half-life of clearance.

All of the patients (see Table 1 for the characteristics of those reported by Sharma et al.[16]) underwent standard 2-dimensional echocardiographic and Doppler flow studies prior to the exercise test, allowing for determination of the degree of left ventricular hypertrophy, as previously described.[20,21]

The exercise tests were performed on a cycle ergometer in the upright position (Ergometrics 800 S, SensorMedics, Yorba Linda, CA or CardiO$_2$, MedGraphics, St. Paul, MN) using a ramp protocol, from a prior control of unloaded cycling, designed to reach the limit of the patient's exercise tolerance in approximately 10 minutes. This required ramp-incremental rates that varied from 5 to 15 W/min based on the patient's account of daily physical activity and also age, gender, and medical history. Although we ensured that the subjects gave a "good" effort (i.e., "can you go for another minute?" repeatedly), we did not coerce the subjects to make "extreme" effort at the limit of tolerance (i.e., "1 more minute!") as we would in the case of an athlete, for example.

During the tests the subjects breathed through a mouthpiece attached to a low dead space and low-resistance flow meter, previously calibrated using a constant 3-L volume input over a wide range of airflow. Respired gas was continuously sampled from the mouthpiece and analyzed for O$_2$ and CO$_2$ using rapidly responding sensors. These were calibrated using precision-analyzed gases. The signals from these devices underwent analog-to-digital conversion for the breath-by-breath determination and display

_____ **Table 1** _____

Characteristics of Patients with Hypertrophic Cardiomyopathy

	Mean	Number	Percentage
Males		80	59%
Females		55	41%
Age (years)	43±15		
Dyspnea:			
New York Heart Association I		62	46%
New York Heart Association II		59	43%
New York Heart Association III		14	10%
Chest pain atypical	20	15%	
exertional	30	22%	
atypical and exertional	6	4%	
Syncope		14	10%
Left ventricular wall thickness (mm)	19±5		
≤12 mm.		9	7%
13-14 mm		20	15%
15-20 mm	66	49%	
21-25 mm		31	23%
>25 mm		9	7%
Magnitude (Wigle score)	4.5±2.6		
Asymmetric hypertrophy		82	65%
Concentric hypertrophy		32	12%
Apical hypertrophy		12	10%
Left ventricular outflow gradient			
<30 mm Hg		96	71%
≥30 mm Hg		39	29%
Left ventricular end-diastolic dimension (mm)	43±6		
Left ventricular end-systolic dimension (mm)	25±1		
Left atrial diameter (mm)	43±8		

Reprinted from American Journal of Cardiology, Vol. 86, No. 2. Sharma et al: Utility of cardiopulmonary exercise, pp. 162-168, 2000, with permission from Excerpta Medica Inc.

of $\dot{V}O_2$, CO_2 output ($\dot{V}CO_2$), ventilation ($\dot{V}E$), and related ventilatory and cardiopulmonary indices, as described by Beaver et al.[22] A 12-lead electrocardiogram was performed in each subject, and selected lead configurations and heart rate (HR) were continuously displayed for observation throughout the test. Blood pressure was determined by auscultation at regular intervals throughout the test. The average $\dot{V}O_2$ over the last 15 seconds was used as an index of the subject's peak $\dot{V}O_2$. The θ_L was estimated not only by the "V-slope" method, as described by Beaver et al.,[23] but also from the profiles of the ventilatory equivalents for CO_2 and O_2 ($\dot{V}E/\dot{V}CO_2$ and $\dot{V}E/\dot{V}O_2$, respectively) and the end-tidal partial pressures of CO_2 and O_2 ($P_{ET}CO_2$ and $P_{ET}O_2$, respectively) as recommended by Whipp et al.[24] (Fig. 1) (i.e., based on the acceleration of $\dot{V}CO_2$ in excess of that derived from aerobic metabolism and which is not attributable to hyperventilation).

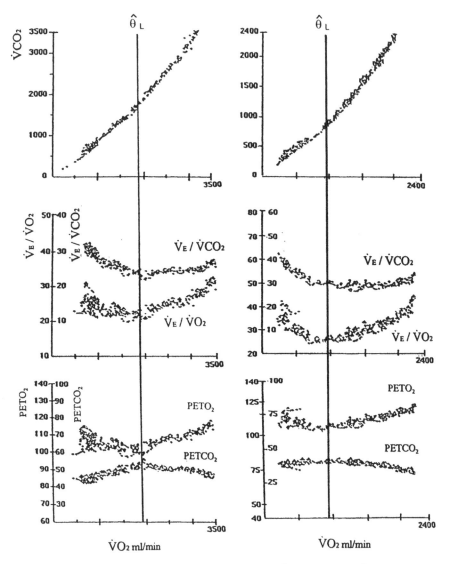

Figure 1. Estimation of the lactate threshold (θ_L) from pulmonary gas exchange responses to rapid incremental cycle ergometer exercise in a representative patient with hypertrophic cardiomyopathy (right) and a control subject (left), as a function of O_2 uptake $(\dot{V}O_2)$: CO_2 output $(\dot{V}CO_2, mL/min)$, ventilatory equivalents for CO_2 and O_2 $(\dot{V}E/\dot{V}CO_2, \dot{V}E/\dot{V}O_2)$, and end-tidal partial pressures of CO_2 and O_2 $(P_{ET}CO_2$ and $P_{ET}O_2$, mm Hg). From Heart 1998;80:60-67, with permission from the BMJ Publishing Group.

The slope of the $\dot{V}O_2$ response as a function of work rate $(\Delta\dot{V}O_2/\Delta WR)$ was determined from the linear phase of the ramp response profile (Fig. 2). The slope of the $\dot{V}E$ response as a function of $\dot{V}CO_2$ $(\Delta\dot{V}E/\Delta\dot{V}CO_2$ slope) was determined over the linear region of the relationship, i.e., prior to the onset of respiratory compensation (Fig. 2). For those cases in which the O_2 pulse

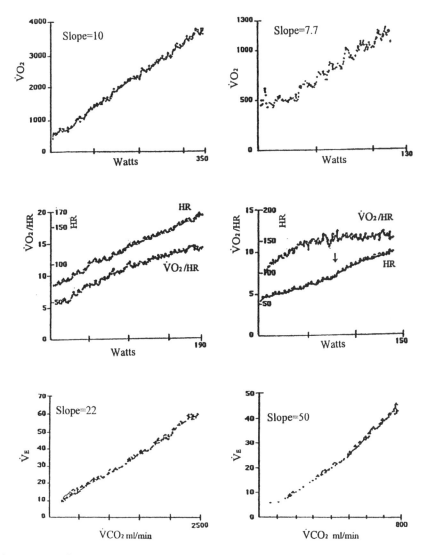

Figure 2. Cardiorespiratory and pulmonary responses to rapid incremental cycle-ergometer exercise in a representative patient with hypertrophic cardiomyopathy ([HCM] right) and a control subject (left). Work rate (watts), heart rate (HR, beats/min), and O_2 pulse ($\dot{V}O_2$/HR, mL O_2/min) as a function of O_2 uptake ($\dot{V}O_2$), and ventilation ($\dot{V}E$, L/min) as a function of CO_2 output ($\dot{V}CO_2$). The arrow on the O_2 pulse-$\dot{V}O_2$ relationship for the HCM patient indicates the onset of flattening (see text for further details). From Heart 1998;80:60-67, with permission from the BMJ Publishing Group.

(i.e., $\dot{V}O_2$/HR) was judged to attain a constant value despite work rate continuing to increase, we ensured that this was not simply an artifact of the low-slope region of a shallow hyperbolic $\dot{V}O_2$/HR profile by verifying that the onset of the constancy coincided with a clear deflection in the HR response, as shown in Figure 2.

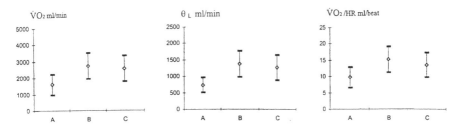

Figure 3. Group-mean (±1 standard deviation) values for peak O_2 uptake ($\dot{V}O_2$), lactate threshold (θ_L), and maximum O_2 pulse in (A) patients with hypertrophic cardiomyopathy, (B) control subjects, and (C) the predicted normal values of Wasserman et al.[10] From Heart 1998;80:60-67, with permission from the BMJ Publishing Group.

As previously shown,[8,9] patients with HCM manifested low exercise tolerance, as reflected by both a low peak $\dot{V}O_2$ and a low θ_L, with an associated reduction in peak $\dot{V}O_2/HR$ (Fig. 3, panels A) compared to either the control group (Fig. 3, panels B) or the predicted values of Wasserman et al.[10] (Fig. 3, panels C).

There was either a very poor relationship or no relationship between the New York Heart Association functional class, the calculated left ventricular outflow gradient, and the maximum left ventricular wall thickness with either the peak or submaximal pulmonary gas exchange indices. Similarly, resting stroke volume proved to be a poor predictive index of these functions. Only the peak $\dot{V}O_2/HR$ was significantly correlated with resting stroke volume, but even here approximately 3-fold variations of resting stroke volume were associated with any given value of the peak $\dot{V}O_2/HR$. The most interesting correlate of peak $\dot{V}O_2$ was shown by Lele et al.[25] to be the time to peak ventricular filling during exercise (Fig. 4), i.e., an index of diastolic function. In contrast, there was no significant relationship between peak $\dot{V}O_2$ and peak exercise ejection fraction. Resting Doppler indices of diastolic function, however, have been shown to be poor predictors of both symptomatic status and maximum exercise tolerance. There was, however, a consistently good and significant relationship between the θ_L, used here as an effort-independent index of exercise tolerance, and the other cardiopulmonary indices determined from the incremental test (Fig. 5). Not surprisingly, the θ_L was highly correlated with both peak $\dot{V}O_2$ and peak $\dot{V}O_2/HR$ (Fig. 5). Interestingly, however, both the $\Delta\dot{V}O_2/\Delta WR$ slope and the $\Delta\dot{V}E/\Delta\dot{V}CO_2$ slope were also significantly correlated with the θ_L, the former positively, and the latter negatively.

In approximately 30% of the patients, $\Delta\dot{V}O_2/\Delta WR$ was abnormally low. Interestingly, in most cases the low slope was evident from the beginning of the exercise test rather than becoming reduced at high work rates, as has been demonstrated in ischemic[10] or chronic heart failure.[26] This slope, however, should be interpreted with caution. It has been demonstrated that the linear $\dot{V}O_2$-work rate relationship during an incremental ramp test can

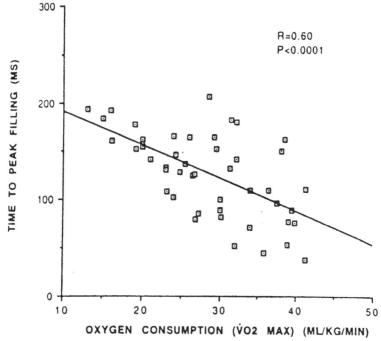

Figure 4. Time to peak ventricular filling during exercise as a function of peak O_2 uptake ($\dot{V}O_2$) in a group of patients with hypertrophic cardiomyopathy. From Lele et al, Exercise capacity in hypertrophic cardiomyopathy. Circulation 1995;92:2886-2894.

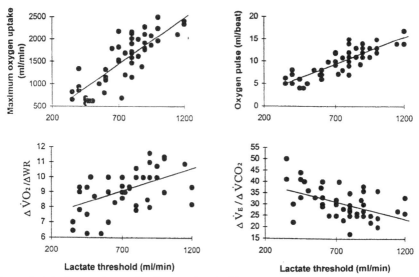

Figure 5. Maximum O_2 uptake, lactate threshold, maximum O_2 pulse, the slope of the linear phase of the $\dot{V}O_2$-work rate relationship ($\Delta\dot{V}O_2/\Delta WR$) (mL O_2/min), and the slope of the linear phase of the $\dot{V}E$-$\dot{V}CO_2$ relationship ($\Delta\dot{V}E/\Delta\dot{V}CO_2$) as a function of the lactate threshold in the hypertrophic cardiomyopathy group. From Heart 1998;80:60-67, with permission from the BMJ Publishing Group.

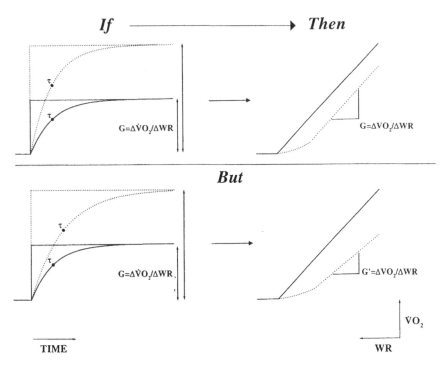

Figure 6. Schematic representation of O_2 uptake ($\dot{V}O_2$) as a function of time in response to moderate intensity, constant load exercise (left) and ramp-incremental exercise (right). For normal subjects (left upper panel), the time constant (τ) of exponential $\dot{V}O_2$ response to the constant load forcing is unaffected by work rate. The equivalent response to the ramp (right upper panel) is a lagged-linear profile whose slope (G) in the linear region = $\Delta\dot{V}O_2/\Delta WR$. The lower panels represent a scenario in which τ becomes longer as work rate increases, but with no change in the steady state gain (G). Interestingly, this predicts that the linear phase of the $\dot{V}O_2$ response to the ramp will increase at a slower rate; i.e., with a low apparent gain. (See text for further details.)

be used as an index of work efficiency in *normal* subjects.[12] This is a necessary consequence of both the time constant and "gain" of the $\dot{V}O_2$ response kinetics being not appreciably different over the range of work rates for which $\dot{V}O_2$ can attain a steady state (see reference 27 for discussion). To our knowledge, however, this has only been established for normal subjects— and certainly not for patients with HCM. Were the time constant for the $\dot{V}O_2$ kinetics to become longer as work rate increases (i.e., consistent with recruitment of muscle fibers less "trained," in the sense that these work rates are not normally encountered during their range of normal physical activity, or as a result of abnormal muscle blood flow or flow distribution), then even if the steady state gain was constant and hence the fundamental steady state efficiency to be unchanged, this would still yield a low apparent gain on the incremental ramp as evident in the $\dot{V}O_2$-work rate relationship (Fig. 6). The low slope of the relationship (i.e., $\Delta\dot{V}O_2/\Delta WR$) would therefore not reflect high efficiency of energy transfer, but rather would be a representation of altered $\dot{V}O_2$ response kinetics. Further work is clearly needed to resolve the mechanism of such low slopes during ramp tests in HCM and also in other cardiopulmonary diseases.

The profile of $\dot{V}O_2/HR$ in patients with HCM is of interest, as the $\dot{V}O_2/HR$ is quantitatively equivalent to the product of the stroke volume and the arterio-mixed venous O_2 content difference. In more than 50% of the patients, the increase in $\dot{V}O_2/HR$ with increasing work rate slowed appreciably or became flat at high work rates (e.g., Fig. 2), such that the further increase in $\dot{V}O_2$ was actually HR dependent. We cannot, from these studies, resolve the mechanism responsible for the flattening of the $\dot{V}O_2/HR$ at high work rates, although an abnormal stroke volume response would be consistent with the cardiac dysfunction, especially since a failure to augment stroke volume during exercise has been previously demonstrated in some patients with HCM.[25,28] However, we cannot naturally rule out from these results that a hyperkinetic cardiac output response[29] or a muscle O_2 extraction defect (coexpressed skeletal myopathies having been demonstrated in HCM patients[30-32]) are not also contributory. The resolution of the proportional contributions requires direct measurement of these variables during the "flattened" phase of the $\dot{V}O_2/HR$ response.

The $\Delta\dot{V}E/\Delta\dot{V}CO_2$ slope during incremental exercise is becoming a widely used index of the "appropriateness" of the $\dot{V}E$ response,[33-36,37] with high slopes thought to be reflective of either a high dead space fraction of the tidal volume (VD/VT) and/or frank hyperventilation (i.e., reduced arterial PCO_2). Others,[10,11,38] however, use $\dot{V}E/\dot{V}CO_2$ at the θ_L for this purpose. It is therefore instructive to consider the differences between these two indices. The linear relationship between $\dot{V}E$ and $\dot{V}CO_2$ can be represented by equation 1:

$$\dot{V}E = m \ \dot{V}CO_2 = c \qquad (1)$$

where m is the $\Delta\dot{V}E/\Delta\dot{V}CO_2$ slope and c is the $\dot{V}E$ intercept. Dividing equation 1 throughout by $\dot{V}CO_2$ yields equation 2:

$$\dot{V}E/\dot{V}CO_2 = m + c/\dot{V}CO_2 \qquad (2)$$

or the slope, m = $\dot{V}E/\dot{V}CO_2 - c/\dot{V}CO_2$

Note here that, as m and c are constants, $\dot{V}E/\dot{V}CO_2$ declines hyperbolically as work rate (and $\dot{V}CO_2$) increases. $\dot{V}E/\dot{V}CO_2$, however, may be represented physiologically, such that $PaCO_2$ and VD/VT now become rigorous determinants of $\dot{V}E/\dot{V}CO_2$, as shown in equation 3:

$$\dot{V}E/\dot{V}CO_2 = 863/\{PaCO_2 \ (1 - VD/VT)\} \qquad (3)$$

where $PaCO_2$ is arterial PCO_2. Consequently, as previously described by Whipp and Wasserman,[39] "the $\dot{V}E-\dot{V}CO_2$ relationship should be described by both its slope and intercept parameters" for rigorous interpretation. However, as $\Delta\dot{V}E/\Delta\dot{V}CO_2$ represents the asymptote of the decreasing $\dot{V}E/\dot{V}CO_2$

Table 2

Number of Abnormal Responses (n=50)					
$\Delta\dot{V}_E/\Delta\dot{V}_{CO_2}$		$\Delta\dot{V}_{O_2}/\Delta WR$		$\dot{V}_{O_2}/HR$	
28		16		27	
$\Delta\dot{V}_{O_2}/\Delta WR$	$\dot{V}_{O_2}/HR$	$\Delta\dot{V}_E/\Delta\dot{V}_{CO_2}$	$\dot{V}_{O_2}/HR$	$\Delta\dot{V}_E/\Delta\dot{V}_{CO_2}$	$\Delta\dot{V}_{O_2}/\Delta WR$
14	21	14	11	21	11
10		10		10	

HR = heart rate; WR = work rate.

profile, poorly fit subjects who begin isocapnic buffering at a relatively low $\dot{V}_{CO_2}$ would therefore have a $\dot{V}_E/\dot{V}_{CO_2}$ at θ_L that is high compared to a fitter subject, despite both having the same $\dot{V}_E/\dot{V}_{CO_2}$ slope. Habedank et al.[35] have demonstrated, using a modified Naughton treadmill exercise test, that the $\Delta\dot{V}_E/\Delta\dot{V}_{CO_2}$ slope increases in normal subjects as a function of age. In a randomized study, Neder et al.[40] have recently also shown this to be the case for ramp-incremental cycle ergometry. Using a value for $\Delta\dot{V}_E/\Delta\dot{V}_{CO_2}$ of 30 as the upper limit of normal, approximately one third of our patients manifested abnormally high slopes. As we did not determine arterial blood gas values in this study, we cannot resolve the mechanism of this high slope; in chronic heart failure, it has been shown to be a consequence of a high V_D/V_T rather than a low $PaCO_2$.[34,36,38,41] Interestingly, the patients with abnormally high $\Delta\dot{V}_E/\Delta\dot{V}_{CO_2}$ did not differ from the controls with respect to either $P_{ET}CO_2$ or breathing pattern, possibly suggesting an increased dead space fraction of the breath resulting from ventilation/perfusion abnormality.

A large proportion of the 50 patients studied by Jones et al.[15] had abnormalities in $\Delta\dot{V}_E/\Delta\dot{V}_{CO_2}$, $\dot{V}_{O_2}/\Delta WR$, and peak $\dot{V}_{O_2}/HR$ (20, 16, and 27, respectively). Table 2 presents the number of patients who had abnormalities in one, two, or all three of these variables; i.e., 10 patients (20%) having abnormal responses of all three indices. What is perhaps most instructive from this table, however, is not that so many patients presented with a single, double, or triple gas exchange abnormality, but that there was a large proportion of patients with known (and often apparently severe) HCM who displayed no discernibly abnormal index of the submaximal gas exchange response profile. It is therefore clear that further understanding of the mechanisms responsible for the reduced exercise tolerance and peak $\dot{V}_{O_2}$ in patients with HCM is likely to require more invasive investigation of both cardiovascular and pulmonary function *during* the exercise.

Summary

Patients with HCM typically manifest exercise intolerance associated with low peak $\dot{V}_{O_2}$ and low θ_L. These characteristics, however, are not discriminatory, also being evident in patients with a wide range of functional abnormalities and even in normal but chronically sedentary subjects. We therefore established the breath-by-breath profile of cardiopulmonary and metabolic responses to ramp-incremental cycle ergometry in a large group of patients with HCM (and age-matched controls) in an attempt to educe more subtle evidence of abnormality that may be pathognomic of HCM.

There was little or no relationship between the New York Heart Association functional class, the estimated left ventricular outflow gradient, or the maximum ventricular wall thickness with either the peak or submaximal pulmonary gas exchange indices. Similarly, resting stroke volume proved to be a poor predictive index of these functions. Only the peak $\dot{V}O_2/HR$ was significantly correlated with resting stroke volume, but even here approximately 3-fold variations of resting stroke volume were associated with any given value of the peak $\dot{V}O_2/HR$. The θ_L was highly correlated (positively) with peak $\dot{V}O_2$, peak $\dot{V}O_2/HR$, and the $\Delta\dot{V}O_2/\Delta WR$ slope; the $\Delta\dot{V}E/\Delta\dot{V}CO_2$ slope and the related $\dot{V}E/\dot{V}CO_2$ were also significantly correlated with the θ_L, but in this case negatively.

A large proportion of the patients studied had abnormalities in $\Delta\dot{V}E/\Delta\dot{V}CO_2$ and $\dot{V}E/\dot{V}CO_2$ (high), $\Delta\dot{V}O_2/\Delta WR$ (low throughout the exercise), and maximum $\dot{V}O_2/HR$ (low and often "flat"), with some 20% having abnormal responses of all three indices. However, what is perhaps most instructive is that such a large proportion of patients with known (and even severe) HCM displayed no discernible abnormality in the submaximal gas exchange response profile. Further understanding of the mechanisms responsible for the reduced exercise tolerance in patients with HCM is likely to require more invasive investigation of both cardiovascular and pulmonary function *during* the exercise.

References

1. Malik MS, Watkins H. The molecular genetics of hypertrophic cardiomyopathy. Curr Opinion Cardiol 1997;12:295-302.

2. Varnava AM, Elliott PM, Baboonian C, Davison F, Davies MJ, McKenna WJ. Hypertrophic cardiomyopathy without hypertrophy: two families with myocardial disarray in the absence of increased myocardial mass. Br Heart J 1990;63:287-290.

3. McKenna W, Deanfield J, Faruqui A, England D, Oakley C, Goodwin J. Prognosis in hypertrophic cardiomyopathy: role of age and clinical, electrocardiographic and hemodynamic features. Am J Cardiol 1981;47:532-538.

4. Elliott PM, Gimeno Blanes JR, Mahon NG, Poloniecki JD, McKenna WJ. Relation between the severity of left ventricular hypertrophy and prognosis in patients with hypertrophic cardiomyopathy. Lancet 2001;357:420-424.

5. Cecchi F, Maron BJ, Epstein SE. Long-term outcome of patients with hypertrophic cardiomyopathy successfully resuscitated after cardiac arrest. J Am Coll Cardiol 1989;13:1283-1288.

6. Frank S, Braunwald E. Idiopathic hypertrophic subaortic stenosis. Clinical analysis of 126 patients with emphasis on the natural history. Circulation 1968;37: 759-788.

7. Chikamori T, Counihan PJ, Doi YL, et al. Mechanisms of exercise limitation in hypertrophic cardiomyopathy. J Am Coll Cardiol 1992;19:507-512.

8. Nihoyannopoulos P, Karatasakis G, Frenneaux M, McKenna WJ, Oakley CM. Diastolic function in hypertrophic cardiomyopathy: relation to exercise capacity. J Am Coll Cardiol 1992;19:536-540.

9. Whyte GP, Sharma S, George K, McKenna WJ. Exercise gas exchange responses in the differentiation of pathologic left ventricular hypertrophy. Med Sci Sports Exerc 1999;31:1237-1241.

10. Wasserman K, Hansen JE, Sue DY, et al. Principles of Exercise Testing and Interpretation. 3rd ed. Philadelphia: Lea & Febiger; 1999.

11. Roca J, Whipp BJ. Clinical Exercise Testing. European Respiratory Monograph. Vol. 2(6). Sheffield, UK: European Respiratory Journals Ltd.; 1997.

12. Whipp BJ, Davis JA, Torres F, Wasserman K. A test to determine parameters of aerobic function during exercise. J Appl Physiol 1981;50:217-221.

13. Buchfuhrer MJ, Hansen JE, Robinson TE, Sue DY, Wasserman K, Whipp BJ. Optimizing the exercise protocol for cardiopulmonary assessment. J Appl Physiol 1983;55:1558-1564.

14. Weisman IM, Zeballos RJ. An integrated approach to the interpretation of cardiopulmonary exercise testing. Clin Chest Med 1994;15:421-445.

15. Jones S, Elliott PM, Sharma S, McKenna WJ, Whipp BJ. Cardiopulmonary response to exercise in patients with hypertrophic cardiomyopathy. Heart 1998; 80:60-67.

16. Sharma S, Elliott P, Whyte G, et al. Utility of cardiopulmonary exercise in the assessment of clinical determinants of functional capacity in hypertrophic cardiomyopathy. Am J Cardiol 2000;86:162-168.

17. WHO/ISFC Task Force. Report of the WHO/ISFC Task Force on the definition and classification of cardiomyopathies. Br Heart J 1980;44:672-673.

18. Watkins H, Rosenzweig A, Hwang DS, et al. Characteristics and prognostic implications of myosin missense mutations in familial hypertrophic cardiomyopathy. N Engl J Med 1992;326:1108-1114.

19. McKenna WJ, Castro Beiras A, Penas Lado M. The cardiomyopathies. Br Heart J 1994;72(suppl):S4-S23.

20. Maron BJ, Gottdiener JS, Epstein SE. Patterns and significance of distribution of left ventricular hypertrophy in hypertrophic cardiomyopathy: a wide-angle two dimensional echocardiographic study of 125 patients. Am J Cardiol 1981;48: 418-428.

21. Shapiro LM, McKenna WJ. Distribution of left ventricular hypertrophy in hypertrophic cardiomyopathy: a two dimensional echocardiographic study of 125 patients. J Am Coll Cardiol 1983;2:437-444.

22. Beaver WL, Wasserman K, Whipp BJ. On-line computer analysis and breath-by-breath graphical display of exercise function tests. J Appl Physiol 1973;34:128-132.

23. Beaver WL, Wasserman K, Whipp BJ. A new method for detecting the anaerobic threshold by gas exchange. J Appl Physiol 1986;60:2020-2027.

24. Whipp BJ, Ward SA, Wasserman K. Respiratory markers of the anaerobic threshold. Adv Cardiol 1986;35:47-64.

25. Lele SS, Thomson HL, Seo H, Belenkie I, McKenna WJ, Frenneaux MP. Exercise capacity in hypertrophic cardiomyopathy. Role of stroke volume limitation, heart rate and diastolic filling characteristics. Circulation 1995;192:2886-2894.

26. Cohen-Solal A. Cardiopulmonary exercise testing in chronic heart failure. In: Wasserman K (ed): Exercise Gas Exchange in Heart Disease. Armonk, NY: Futura Publishing Co.; 1996:17-35.

27. Whipp BJ, Ozyener F. The kinetics of exertional O_2 uptake: assumptions and inferences. Med della Sport 1998;51:39-49.

28. Losse B, Kuhn H, Loogen F, Schulte HD. Exercise performance in hypertrophic cardiomyopathies. Eur Heart J 1983;4(suppl F):197-208.

29. Counihan PJ, Frenneaux MP, Webb DJ, McKenna WJ. Abnormal vascular responses to supine exercise in hypertrophic cardiomyopathy. Circulation 1991; 84:686-696.

30. Cuda G, Fananapazir L, Zhu WS, Sellers JR, Epstein ND. Skeletal muscle expression and abnormal function of β myosin in hypertrophic cardiomyopathy. J Clin Invest 1993;91:2861-2865.

31. Lankford EB, Fananapazir L, Sweeney HL. Abnormal contractile properties of muscle fibres expressing beta-myosin heavy chain gene mutations in patients with hypertrophic cardiomyopathy. J Clin Invest 1995;95:1409-1412.

32. Caforio AL, Rossi B, Risaliti R, et al. Type 1 fiber abnormalities in skeletal muscle of patients with hypertrophic and dilated cardiomyopathy: evidence of subclinical myogenic myopathy. J Am Coll Cardiol 1989;14:1464-1473.

33. Clark AJ, Volterrani M, Swan JW, Coats AJ. The increased ventilatory response to exercise in chronic heart failure: relation to pulmonary pathology. Heart 1997;77:138-146.

34. Buller NP, Poole-Wilson PA. Mechanism of the increased ventilatory response to exercise in patients with chronic heart failure. Br Heart J 1990;63:281-283.

35. Habedank D, Reindl I, Vietzke G, et al. Ventilatory efficiency and exercise tolerance in 101 healthy volunteers. Eur J Appl Physiol 1998;77:421-426.

36. Metra, M, Raccagni D, Carini G, et al. Ventilatory and arterial blood gas changes during exercise in heart failure. In: Wasserman K (ed): Exercise Gas Exchange in Heart Disease. Armonk, NY: Futura Publishing Co.; 1996:125-143.

37. Clark AJ, Volterrani M, Swan JW, Coats AJ. Ventilation-perfusion mismatch in chronic heart failure. Int J Cardiol 1995;48:138-146.

38. Lewis DA, Sietsema KE, Casaburi R, Sue DY. Inaccuracy of noninvasive estimates of VD/VT in clinical exercise testing. Chest 1994;106:1476-1480.

39. Whipp BJ, Wasserman K. Exercise. In Murray JF, Nadel JA (eds): Textbook of Respiratory Medicine. Philadelphia: W.B. Saunders Co.; 1994:236.

40. Neder JA, Nery LA, Peres C, Whipp BJ. Reference values for dynamic responses to incremental cycle ergometry in males and females aged 20 to 80. Am J Respir Crit Care Med 2001;15:1481-1486.

41. Banning AP, Lewis NP, Northridge DB, Elborn JS, Hendersen AH. Perfusion ventilation mismatch during exercise in chronic heart failure—an investigation of circulatory determinants. Br Heart J 1995;74:27-33.

12

Oxygen Uptake Abnormalities During Exercise in Coronary Artery Disease

Haruki Itoh, MD, Akihiko Tajima, BS,
Akira Koike, MD, Naohiko Osada, MD,
Tomoko Maeda, BS, Makoto Kato, MD,
Kazuto Omiya, MD, Long Tai Fu, MD,
Hiroshi Watanabe, MD, and
Kazuzo Kato, MD

Although exercise electrocardiography is widely used as a screening examination for coronary artery disease (CAD), it does not detect all CAD and results are sometimes abnormal despite the absence of CAD.[1] When myocardial work is increased so that there is an O_2 supply/O_2 requirement imbalance in the ischemic area of the myocardium, abnormal wall motion develops in the ischemic area of the left ventricle.[2] Thus, the increase in cardiac output as exercise intensity increases would be expected to be attenuated. Since O_2 uptake ($\dot{V}O_2$) is determined by cardiac output times the arterial-venous O_2 difference, we hypothesized that the change in cardiac output caused by ischemia will affect $\dot{V}O_2$ kinetics and the change in $\dot{V}O_2$ relative to change in work rate ($\Delta\dot{V}O_2/\Delta WR$) at the level of $\dot{V}O_2$ at which ischemia-induced myocardial dyskinesis develops. From this theoretical perceptive, we investigated the $\Delta\dot{V}O_2/\Delta WR$ change during incremental exercise in patients with suspected CAD based on an exercise stress test, limited to electrocardiographic measurements, conducted previously.

From Wasserman K (ed): *Cardiopulmonary Exercise Testing and Cardiovascular Health.* Armonk, NY: Futura Publishing Company, Inc.; © 2002.

Methods

The study comprised 26 patients who had anginalike symptoms and exhibited significant ST depression of more than 1 mm during an exercise test. The patients were all male, aged 61 ± 9 (mean$\pm$SD) years. Those with myocardial disease, atrial fibrillation, lung disease, and heart failure were excluded.

Symptom-limited exercise testing with a cycle ergometer was performed using the CPE-2000 (MedGraphics, St. Paul, MN) with expired gas analysis. We employed a ramp protocol consisting of a 0-W warm-up for 4 minutes followed by a 1-W increase every 6 seconds until the patient showed exhaustion, ST depression of more than 2 mm, serious arrhythmia, or abnormal blood pressure response. Gas exchange analysis was performed on a breath-by-breath basis using an Aeromonitor AE-280 (Minato Ikagaku, Osaka, Japan), and all the plots were converted into time domain data for every 3 seconds. $\dot{V}O_2$ data were smoothed by an 8-point moving average, and the $\Delta\dot{V}O_2/\Delta WR$ was derived by linear regression of the $\dot{V}O_2$ plots.

A Stress Test System ML-5000 (Fukuda Denshi, Tokyo, Japan) was used to monitor the heart rate (HR) and ST level, at 40 ms from the J-point in the lead of the 12-lead electrocardiogram that showed the most prominent change in ST level, throughout the test. We determined the point of 1-mm ST depression (ST-Dep) by the ST level trendgram and then derived the $\Delta\dot{V}O_2/\Delta WR$ during the 2-minute period before and after the onset of ST-Dep during exercise.

We calculated the ratio of $\Delta\dot{V}O_2/\Delta WR$ above the ST-Dep over that below the ST-Dep ($\Delta\dot{V}O_2$ slope ratio) as an index for the change in $\dot{V}O_2$ kinetics. Peak $\dot{V}O_2$ was defined as the average of $\dot{V}O_2$ during the last 30 seconds of the exercise tests, and anaerobic threshold (AT) was determined using criteria proposed by Wasserman and McIlroy.[3] The O_2 pulse ($\dot{V}O_2/HR$) during exercise was also calculated as a parameter for stroke volume.

All patients underwent coronary angiography and were classified into three groups based on the number of lesions with significant stenosis (>75%): patients with normal coronary arteries (0VD), those with single vessel disease (SVD), and those with multivessel disease (MVD). The criteria for evaluation of significant stenosis were based on the American Heart Association Committee Report on diagnosis of CAD.[4] When patients showed normal coronary arteries, the provocation test for vasospasm using acetylcholine was done. Patients diagnosed with vasospastic angina pectoris were excluded.

Statistical Analysis

The mean values of parameters in the three groups were compared by analysis of variance. A value of $p < 0.05$ was considered significant. Data are expressed as mean$\pm$SD.

_____ Table 1 _____

Baseline Physical Characteristics in Angiographically Based Coronary Artery Disease Study Groups

Patient group	OVD	SVD	MVD
No. of case (n)	8	7	8
Height (cm)	164.0±5.0	167±5.6	166±3.1
Weight (kg)	70.2±9.6	67.1±7.9	68.9±7.7
Age (years)	56.8±5.1	65.7±9.7	59.5±8.0
Hemoglobin (g/dL)	15.6±5.1	14.1±1.1	14.7±1.9
LVEF (%)	74.1±6.2	70.7±7.9	65.1±9.9*
No. of diseased vessels	0	1	2.8±0.5

OVD = zero vessel disease; LVEF = left ventricular ejection fraction measured by echocardiography; MVD = multivessel disease; SVD = single vessel disease. *p<0.05 versus OVD and SVD.

Results

Three of 26 patients were excluded from the analysis because of positive acetylcholine test without significant organic stenosis in the coronary arteries. The profiles of the remaining patients are presented in Table 1. The only statistical difference in the patient backgrounds among the three groups was a significantly lower left ventricular ejection fraction in the MVD group; however, this parameter was still within normal limits in this group.

Endpoint of Exercise Test and Exercise Time

The endpoint of the exercise test is shown in Table 2. All of the patients in the OVD group stopped the exercise test because of leg fatigue. In contrast, 3 of 7 patients in the SVD group and 7 of 8 patients in the MVD group stopped the test because of either chest pain or ST depression of more than 2 mm. The exercise time including warm-up was 678±110, 547±73, and 536±123 seconds in the OVD, SVD, and MVD groups, respectively.

_____ Table 2 _____

Factors Determining Endpoint of Exercise Test in Angiographically Divided Patient Groups

Patient group	OVD	SVD	MVD
Chest pain	0	1	4
ST depression	0	2	3
Leg fatigue, SOB	8	4	1

OVD = zero vessel disease; MVD = multivessel disease; SOB = shortness of breath; SVD = single vessel disease.

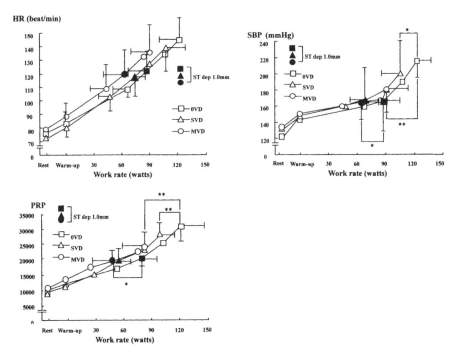

Figure 1. Heart rate (HR), systolic blood pressure (SBP), and pressure-rate product (PRP) during exercise test. Data are plotted at rest, warm-up, 2 minutes before 1 mm of ST depression, 1-mm ST depression point, and 2 minutes after 1-mm ST depression point. ST-Dep = point of 1 mm ST depression during exercise test. Adapted from Tajima A et al. Shinzo 35(5), with permission.

HR, Systolic Blood Pressure, and Pressure-Rate Product

Figure 1 shows the HR, systolic blood pressure, and pressure-rate product (PRP) during the exercise test. There were no statistical differences among the groups in HR and PRP at rest, during warm-up, and at the ST-Dep point. On the other hand, HR and PRP at peak exercise were higher in the OVD group than in the SVD and MVD groups ($p<0.05$).

AT, Peak $\dot{V}o_2$ and $\dot{V}o_2$/HR

ATs in OVD, SVD, and MVD were 12.9 ± 2.1, 12.2 ± 1.6, and 12.7 ± 1.6 mL/kg/min, respectively (Fig. 2). There was no statistical difference among the groups; however, average peak $\dot{V}o_2$ was higher in the OVD group (24.2 ± 4.2 mL/kg/min) than in the other two groups (SVD: 19.6 ± 3.0 mL/kg/min, MVD: 19.6 ± 3.1 mL/kg/min) (Fig. 2), mainly because of the higher

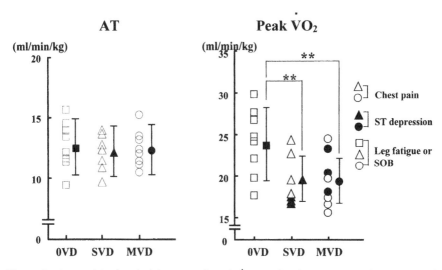

Figure 2. Anaerobic threshold (AT) and peak V̇O₂ in the three groups of patients with ST segment depression divided according to the number of vessels with clinically significant stenosis. There was no difference among AT values in the three groups while peak V̇O₂ decreased along with the severity of the coronary disease. SOB = shortness of breath. Adapted from Tajima A et al. Shinzo 35(5), with permission.

work rate performed. The similar *AT* values indicate that the patients in the three groups had the same level of activities of daily living.

The V̇O₂/HR (stroke volume times arterial-venous O_2 difference) was similar in the three groups at rest and at warm-up, at a time that ischemic changes were not provoked, but it increased less the greater the disease, at the higher work rates (Fig. 3).

V̇O₂ Kinetics Change

Table 3 shows ΔV̇O₂/ΔWR below and above ST-Dep for the three groups. The ΔV̇O₂/ΔWR values were similar below ST-Dep, while the ΔV̇O₂/ΔWR decreased significantly in the MVD group, above ST-Dep. The V̇O₂ slope ratios differ significantly in the three groups (Fig. 4).

Discussion

Hansen et al.[5] reported that ΔV̇O₂/ΔWR increased linearly during the ramp test in normal subjects, while it decreased in patients with pulmonary vascular disease and CAD. This decrease is thought to reflect the insufficiency of oxygen transport to the peripheral tissue. The failure of V̇O₂ to increase appropriately with the work rate is commonly seen in patients with heart failure. This phenomenon reflects the failure for cardiac output (oxygen

O₂ pulse

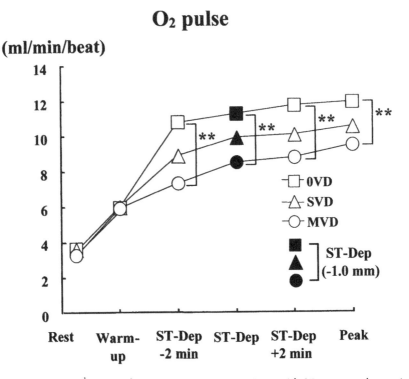

Figure 3. O₂ pulse (V̇O₂/HR) during exercise test in patients with ST segment depression divided into groups according to the number of vessels with clinically significant stenosis. OVD = zero vessel disease; SVD = single vessel disease; MVD = multivessel disease; ST-Dep = point of 1 mm ST depression during exercise test. Adapted from Tajima A et al. Shinzo 35(5), with permission.

flow) to increase appropriately during exercise to meet the muscle O₂ requirement of the work rate.

Although decreased $\Delta\dot{V}O_2/\Delta WR$ is noted even below AT for low or moderate exercise intensity in heart failure patients,[6] the $\Delta\dot{V}O_2/\Delta WR$ decreased only above the ST-Dep point in CAD. In this study, no patient had

___ **Table 3** ___

$\Delta\dot{V}O_2/\Delta WR$ Below and Above ST-Dep Point in Three Angiographically Divided Patient Groups with ST Segment Depression in Response to an Electrocardiographic Stress Test

Group	$\Delta\dot{V}O_2/\Delta WR$ below ST-Dep	$\Delta\dot{V}O_2/\Delta WR$ above ST-Dep
OVD	11.9±1.2	12.7±1.7
SVD	11.5±0.6	10.1±1.7
MVD	11.2±1.1	7.9±2.1*

OVD = zero vessel disease; SVD = single vessel disease; MVD = multivessel disease; ST-Dep = point of 1 mm ST depression during exercise test in all patients; WR = work rate. *p<0.05 versus OVD.

$\Delta \dot{V}O_2 / \Delta WR(\Delta \dot{V}O_2$ slope ratios)

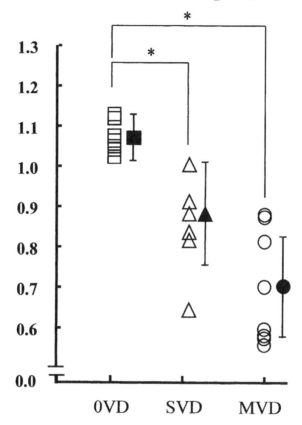

Figure 4. $\Delta \dot{V}_{O_2}$ slope ratios (the ratio of $\Delta \dot{V}_{O_2}/\Delta WR$ above the point of ST-Dep to $\Delta \dot{V}_{O_2}/\Delta WR$ below the point of ST-Dep) in patients with ST segment depression divided into groups according to the number of vessels with clinically significant occlusions. 0VD = zero vessel disease; SVD = single vessel disease; MVD = multivessel disease. Adapted from Tajima A et al. Shinzo 35(5), with permission.

signs or symptoms of heart failure, and there were no differences in *AT* among the three groups, despite the decrease of this parameter in accordance with severity of heart failure.[7] These findings support the conjecture that the decrease of $\Delta \dot{V}_{O_2}/\Delta WR$ during exercise in CAD is due to the change in cardiac performance caused by myocardial ischemic change.

The $\dot{V}_{O_2}/HR$, a parameter for stroke volume, did not differ among the three groups at rest and during warm-up, but it increased less at higher exercise intensities, the extent corresponding to the number of coronary lesions. In fact, we found that the $\dot{V}_{O_2}/HR$ was lower in the SVD and MVD groups than in the 0VD group even at 2 minutes before the ST-Dep point (Fig. 3). This was compatible with a former report[8] that demonstrated an early appearance of mechanical abnormality before electrographic change during incremental exercise in patients with CAD. These findings suggest that once the regional myocardial ischemia is provoked, the pumping function is disturbed, thereby reducing stroke volume and attenuating the increase of the cardiac output. This is consistent with the reduction in the $\dot{V}_{O_2}$ slope, resulting in a low $\Delta\dot{V}_{O_2}/\Delta WR$ above the exercise level at which ST depression develops.

Summary

$\dot{V}_{O_2}$ kinetics changed when regional myocardial ischemia was provoked in CAD. Presumably the change is consequent to the impaired increase in the cardiac output as work rate is increased. This phenomenon may be useful in differentiating false-positive from true-positive electrocardiographic changes obtained during exercise testing for CAD.

References

1. Gianrossi R, Detrano R, Mulvihill D, et al. Exercise-induced ST depression in the diagnosis of coronary artery disease: a meta-analysis. Circulation 1989;80:87-98.
2. Jengo JA, Oren V, Conant R, et al. Effects of maximal exercise stress on left ventricular function in patients with coronary artery disease using first pass radionuclide angiography: a rapid, noninvasive technique for determining ejection fraction and segmental wall motion. Circulation 1979;59:60-65.
3. Wasserman K, McIlroy MB. Detecting the threshold of anaerobic metabolism in cardiac patients during exercise. Am J Cardiol 1964;14:844-852.
4. Austen WG, Edwards JE, Frye RL, et al. A reporting system on patients evaluated for coronary artery disease. Report of the Ad Hoc Committee for Grading of Coronary Artery Disease, Council on Cardiovascular Surgery, American Heart Association. Circulation 1975;51(4 suppl):5-40.
5. Hansen J, Sue DY, Oren A, Wasserman K. Relation of oxygen uptake to work rate in normal men and men with circulatory disorders. Am J Cardiol 1987;59:669-674.
6. Itoh H, Nakamura M, Ikeda C, et al. Changes in oxygen uptake-work rate relationship as a compensatory mechanism in patients with heart failure. Jpn Circ J 1992;56:504-508.
7. Itoh H, Taniguchi K, Koike A, Doi M. Evaluation of severity of heart failure using ventilatory gas analysis. Circulation 1990;81(suppl II):II-31-II-37.
8. Upton MT, Rerych SK, Newman GE, Port S, Cobb FR, Jones RH. Detecting abnormalities in left ventricular function during exercise before angina and ST-segment depression. Circulation 1980;62:341-349.

13

Cardiopulmonary Exercise Testing in Pulmonary Vascular Disease:

Arterial and End-Tidal CO_2 Partial Pressures in Patients with Acute and Chronic Pulmonary Embolism and Primary Pulmonary Hypertension

Peer E. Waurick, MD and Franz X. Kleber, MD, PhD

The lungs, in addition to functioning as an oxygenator and blood filter, play a dominant role in achieving acid-base balance by excreting carbon dioxide, thereby helping to maintain an optimal blood pH. Normally, the pulmonary vascular bed allows a broad range of flows while offering remarkably little resistance. Pulmonary hypertension results when reductions in the caliber of the pulmonary vessels and/or increases in pulmonary blood flow occur.[1] Diseases of the pulmonary circulation, such as acute (a) or chronic (c) pulmonary embolism [(PE); aPE, cPE, respectively] and primary pulmonary hypertension (PPH), characteristically cause reduced perfusion to ventilated alveoli.[2] The matching of ventilation to perfusion of the lungs is an important determinant of ventilatory efficiency and it is known that ventilatory efficiency correlates to the pulmonary artery pressure (PAP) at rest.[3,4] However, the effect of pulmonary hypertension of different etiologies on arterial CO_2 partial pressure ($PaCO_2$), end-tidal CO_2 partial pressure ($PETCO_2$), and arterial end-tidal CO_2 difference [$P(a-ET)CO_2$] have not been systematically investigated and data on these measurements are rare. We

From Wasserman K (ed): *Cardiopulmonary Exercise Testing and Cardiovascular Health.* Armonk, NY: Futura Publishing Company, Inc.; © 2002.

therefore studied $PaCO_2$ and $PetCO_2$ at rest in patients with aPE and cPE and PPH. We also compared these data with PAPs and ventilatory efficiency on exercise ($\dot{V}E$ vs. $\dot{V}CO_2$ slope, over the linear range of the relationship, i.e., before the onset of ventilatory compensation for the exercise metabolic acidosis).

Methods

Patients

We analyzed the $PaCO_2$ and $PetCO_2$ of 54 patients with aPE (25 males, 29 females, mean age 62.4 years, range 23 to 89 years), 23 patients with cPE (12 males, 11 females, mean age 57.5 years, range 22 to 81 years), and 14 patients with PPH (7 males, 7 females, mean age 46.3 years, range 18 to 80 years). In 29 patients with aPE, measurements of $P(a\text{-}ET)CO_2$ were repeated at 1 week, and in 6 patients at 6 months after anticoagulant and/or thrombolytic therapy.

PE was defined as acute in patients with typical symptoms within the past 4 weeks. Case histories with symptoms longer than 4 weeks were defined as cPE. All patients with aPE were recruited in the emergency room and/or in the intensive care unit, while patients with cPE and PPH were treated on an outpatient basis or admitted for elective diagnosis and treatment. The diagnosis was confirmed or ruled out with spiral computed tomography and/or angiography in all patients.

The diagnosis of PPH was established on the basis of a mean PAP of >30 mm Hg and the exclusion of secondary causes of pulmonary hypertension according to the diagnostic criteria reported by Rich et al.[5]

Measurement of $PaCO_2$ and $PetCO_2$ at Rest and Ventilatory Efficiency ($\dot{V}E$ vs. $\dot{V}CO_2$ Slope) During Exercise

In all patients with aPE, we measured $PetCO_2$ at rest using portable cardiopulmonary exercise testing (CPET) equipment (Cosmed K4b[2], Cosmed Ltd., Rome, Italy) or the CO_2 detector of the Kion ventilator (Siemens AG, Munich, Germany). Both measure $PetCO_2$ by infrared spectroscopy. Gas was sampled with a tight mask during 2 minutes of breathing at rest. An arterial sample was taken simultaneously for blood gas measurements.

Measurements in patients with cPE and PPH were performed with a Ganshorn cardiopulmonary exercise system (Ganshorn Medizin Electronic GmbH, Niederlauer, Germany). The patients were tested with the modified Naughton protocol[6] on a treadmill. This protocol starts after a 2-minute rest period, followed by incremental exercise with stages of 2 minutes and increments in both slope and velocity of the treadmill. This causes an increment in work rate of about 1 metabolic equivalent (or 3.5 mL O$_2$ kg^{-1} min^{-1}) per stage.

In this study we analyzed PaCO$_2$ and PETCO$_2$ during rest before the start of exercise. The ventilatory efficiency during exercise was assessed by plotting minute ventilation ($\dot{V}$E) against carbon dioxide output ($\dot{V}$CO$_2$), revealing a linear relationship up to the ventilatory compensation point. The slope of this regression represents the ventilatory efficiency during submaximal exercise. Blood was sampled for blood gas measurement from the hyperemic earlobe at rest and for anaerobic threshold during CPET.

P(a-ET)CO$_2$ was calculated as follows:

$$P(a\text{-}ET)CO_2 = (PaCO_2) - (PETCO_2)$$

Measurements of PAP

In all patients with aPE, we performed transthoracic echocardiography in the emergency room and/or in the intensive care unit. The PAPs were calculated by Doppler-derived tricuspid regurgitant peak flow velocity. In patients with aPE, PAP was calculated only by echo, while in patients with cPE and PPH *mean* PAP was measured by right heart catheterization.

Patients with cPE and PPH underwent right heart catheterization to measure systolic, diastolic, and mean PAPs.

Evaluation of PE

To confirm or rule out PE, spiral computed tomography using iohexol as contrast medium was performed in all patients. Pulmonary angiography in aPE was reserved for patients in whom spiral computed tomography remained indeterminate. Patients with cPE and PPH underwent both spiral computed tomography and pulmonary angiography.

Statistical Analysis

All variables are presented as mean±SD.

Results

The results of measurements of PaCO$_2$, PETCO$_2$, and PAP at rest in aPE, cPE, and PPH, and $\dot{V}$E vs $\dot{V}$CO$_2$ slope in cPE and PPH during exercise, are

Table 1

Resting Arterial and End-Tidal CO_2 Tensions, Pulmonary Artery Pressures, and $\dot{V}E$ vs. $\dot{V}CO_2$ Slopes as Measure of Ventilatory Efficiency

	$PaCO_2$ (mm Hg)	$PETCO_2$ (mm Hg)	$P_{(a\text{-}ET)}CO_2$ (mm Hg)	PAP (mm Hg)	$\dot{V}E$ vs. $\dot{V}CO_2$ slope
aPE (n=54)	37.5±8.1	23.6±9.7	13.7±7.5	44.1±14.6*	—
cPE (n=23)	33.6±5.6	25.8±5.7	7.7±3.5	47.4±16.5	49.9±14.4
PPH (n=14)	30.6±4.2	25.4±4.3	3.9±3.2	65.4±19.3	54.6±15.1

aPE = acute pulmonary embolism; cPE = chronic pulmonary embolism; PAP = pulmonary artery pressure; PPH = primary pulmonary hypertension. *Calculated by echo.

shown in Table 1. Patients with aPE had marked elevation in average $P(a\text{-}ET)CO_2$ as a result of decreased $PETCO_2$, but normal $PaCO_2$ values. All three groups had similar $PETCO_2$ values. In both cPE and PPH, values of $PaCO_2$ were below normal (normal value at sea level in adult men: 36 to 42 mm Hg). In cPE, $P(a\text{-}ET)CO_2$ values were higher than in PPH (7.7 vs. 3.9 mm Hg). In both cPE and PPH, patients had similarly elevated $\dot{V}E$ vs. $\dot{V}CO_2$ slopes.

Discussion

Changes in cardiovascular and respiratory function caused by pulmonary vascular diseases are complex and multifactorial. Both the magnitude and the absence or presence of preexisting cardiopulmonary and/or pulmonary diseases are responsible for the hemodynamic and ventilatory consequences in PE.[7] In pulmonary vascular disease, ventilatory impairments may result from ventilation/perfusion mismatching, shunting within the lung consequent to the opening of preexisting pulmonary arterial-venous anastomoses or to a patent foramen ovale, decreased cardiac output, or altered diffusion properties within the lung. Probably these various mechanisms interact and make the understanding of pathophysiology in these diseases difficult.[7]

The most important findings of our study are the comparisons of ventilatory efficiency at rest among three clinical disorders involving the pulmonary circulation, aPE, cPE, and PPH. Reduced ventilatory efficiency in all of these pulmonary vascular diseases is well known and has been described by several authors.[3,4,8-10] Increased dead space ventilation results in a positive $P(a\text{-}ET)CO_2$.[2] This measurement is used as a relatively noninvasive alternative to pulmonary angiography for evaluating and monitoring emergent and critically ill patients suffering aPE.[11-15]

Breen et al.[16,17] described measurements of $PaCO_2$ and $PETCO_2$ in 5 dogs with experimental reversible occluded pulmonary arteries. In their study, by 1 minute after right pulmonary artery occlusion, $PETCO_2$ decreased from 28.7±4.2 to 21.8±3.3 mm Hg[16] and increased immediately after reperfusion from 25 ± 5 to 33 ± 5 mm Hg.[17] These data are comparable to our clinical experience and in agreement with the findings of several studies.[12-15] All of these studies have shown that the relationship between $PaCO_2$ and $P_{ET}CO_2$ is a reliable and rapidly obtainable measurement for diagnosing and monitoring aPE.

There is a paucity of follow-up studies describing disturbances of $PaCO_2$ and $P_{ET}CO_2$ in patients with cPE and/or aPE in the current literature. Wiegand et al.[14] analyzed 12 patients with aPE before and after thrombolytic therapy. They found a decrease of $P(a\text{-}ET)CO_2$ from 9.8 ± 4.5 mm Hg to 2.8 ± 0.9 mm Hg after thrombolytic therapy in these patients. An analysis of our own data did not show as good results. We obtained, in agreement with Wiegand et al.,[14] a marked decrease (average 5.5 mm Hg; data not shown) of $P(a\text{-}ET)CO_2$ 1 week after thrombolytic therapy. We found much lower values for $P(a\text{-}ET)CO_2$ in patients with cPE than in those with aPE.

In patients with PPH, our data confirmed well known resting hyperventilation,[8,18] which seems to be the dominant mechanism of an increased $\dot{V}E$ vs. $\dot{V}CO_2$ slope in PPH.[3] $P(a\text{-}ET)CO_2$ is normally negative.[2] It has, however, been found to be positive in PPH and cPE, but more so in the latter (3.9 ± 3.2 vs. 7.7 ± 3.5). An increased $P(a\text{-}ET)CO_2$ has been shown to correlate with an elevated dead space ventilation.[19] Thus, we postulate that the increase in $\dot{V}E$ vs. $\dot{V}CO_2$ slope is due to ventilation/perfusion mismatch and hyperventilation in cPE and PPH.

Summary

CPET is clinically very helpful in understanding the underlying pathophysiology in pulmonary vascular disease of various causes. PPH and cPE cause similar disturbances of ventilatory efficiency ($\dot{V}E$ vs. $\dot{V}CO_2$ slope). In cPE and PPH, $\dot{V}E$ vs. $\dot{V}CO_2$ slope increases because of ventilation/perfusion mismatch and hyperventilation. In contrast, patients with aPE have a much higher $P(a\text{-}ET)CO_2$, documenting a greater increase in dead space ventilation.

We conclude that $P(a\text{-}ET)CO_2$ is a reliable, noninvasive measurement that is useful for diagnosing aPE in the emergency room setting and for monitoring follow-up in patients with PE. We believe that CPET parameters should be further evaluated as a screening test for detecting pulmonary vascular diseases such as PE and PPH.

Acknowledgment: The authors are indebted to Karlman Wasserman for his advice and encouragement during the performance of the tests and his helpful comments in improving the manuscript.

References

1. Grossman W, Braunwald E. Pulmonary hypertension. In: Braunwald E (ed): Heart Disease: A Textbook of Cardiovascular Medicine. 4th ed. Philadelphia: W.B. Saunders Co.; 1992:790-803.

2. Wasserman K, Hansen JE, Sue DY, et al. Pulmonary vascular disease. In: Principles of Exercise Testing and Interpretation. 3rd ed. Philadelphia: Lippincott Williams & Wilkins; 1999:102-104.

3. Reybrouck T, Mertens L, Schulze-Neick, et al. Ventilatory efficiency for carbon dioxide during exercise in patients with pulmonary hypertension. Clin Physiol 1998;18:337-334.

4. Reindl I, Wernecke KD, Opitz C, et al. Impaired ventilatory efficiency in chronic heart failure: Possible role of pulmonary vasoconstriction. Am Heart J 1998;136:778-785.

5. Rich S, Dantzker DR, Ayres SM, et al. Primary pulmonary hypertension. A national prospective study. Ann Intern Med 1987;107:216-223.

6. Weber KT, Kinasewitz GT, Janicki JS, Fishman AP. Oxygen utilization and ventilation during exercise in patients with chronic heart failure. Circulation 1982;65:1213-1223.

7. Torbicki A, van Beek EJR, Charbonnier B, et al. Guidelines on diagnosis and management of acute pulmonary embolism. Eur Heart J 2000;21:1301-1336.

8. D'Alonzo GE, Gianotti LA, Pohil RL, et al. Comparison of progressive exercise performance of normal subjects and patients with primary pulmonary hypertension. Chest 1987;92:57-62.

9. Dantzker DR, Bower JS. Mechanisms of gas exchange abnormality in patients with chronic obliterative pulmonary vascular disease. J Clin Invest 1979;64:1050-1055.

10. Dantzker DR, D'Alonzo GE, Bower JS, Popat K, Crevey BJ. Pulmonary gas exchange during exercise in patients with chronic obliterative pulmonary hypertension. Am Rev Respir Dis 1984;130:412-416.

11. Levine RL, Wayne MA, Miller CC. End-tidal carbon dioxide and outcome of out-of-hospital cardiac arrest. N Engl J Med 1997;337:301-306.

12. Johanning JM, Veverka TJ, Bays RA, Tong GK, Schmiege SK. Evaluation of suspected pulmonary embolism utilizing end-tidal CO_2 and D-dimer. Am J Surg 1999;178:98-102.

13. Ward KR, Yealy DM. End-tidal carbon dioxide monitoring in emergency medicine, Part 2: Clinical applications. Acad Emerg Med 1998;5:637-646.

14. Wiegand UK, Kurowski V, Giannitsis E, Katus HA, Djonlagic H. Effectiveness of end-tidal carbon dioxide tension for monitoring thrombolytic therapy in acute pulmonary embolism. Crit Care Med 2000;28:3588-3592.

15. Taniguchi S, Irita K, Sakaguchi Y, Takahashi S. Arterial to end-tidal CO_2 gradient as an indicator of silent pulmonary embolism. Lancet 1996;348:1451.

16. Breen PH, Mazumdar B, Skinner SC. How does experimental pulmonary embolism decrease CO_2 elimination. Respir Physiol 1996;105:217-224.

17. Breen PH, Mazumdar B, Skinner SC. Carbon dioxide elimination measures resolution of experimental pulmonary embolus in dogs. Anesth Analg 1996;83:247-253.

18. Theodore J, Robin ED, Morris A, et al. Augmented ventilatory response to exercise pulmonary hypertension. Chest 1986;89:39-44.

19. Ting H, Sun X-G, Chuang ML, Lewis DA, Hansen JE, Wasserman K. A noninvasive assessment of pulmonary perfusion abnormality in patients with primary pulmonary hypertension. Chest 2001;119:824-832.

Abnormalities in Exercise Gas Exchange in Primary Pulmonary Hypertension

Ronald J. Oudiz, MD and Xing-Guo Sun, MD

Primary pulmonary hypertension (PPH) is a disease of the pulmonary vasculature of unknown etiology, with an occurrence of approximately 1 to 2 new cases per million persons per year in the US.[1] A recent rise in the number of cases of PPH resulted from the use of anorexic agents.[2] The most common and often the earliest symptoms of PPH are dyspnea and fatigue.[3]

The underlying pathophysiology in PPH is that of an intrinsic abnormality of the pulmonary vasculature involving intimal fibrosis, medial hypertrophy, and the formation of plexiform lesions. This "vasculopathy" leads to increased pulmonary vascular resistance and failure to perfuse ventilated lung tissue. This ultimately leads to decreased perfusion of the pulmonary vascular bed which, in turn, results in an insufficient increase in cardiac output during exercise.

Several mechanisms are important in inducing dyspnea and fatigue with exercise in patients with PPH. A major factor is that O_2 delivery to skeletal muscles fails to increase normally in response to exercise because pulmonary blood flow, and therefore left ventricular output, does not increase appropriately. In patients with pulmonary vascular disease, cardiac output, and therefore O_2 uptake ($\dot{V}O_2$), does not increase in response to exercise at a rate sufficient to meet the demands of cellular respiration.[4,5] The reason for the inadequate O_2 transport is that the right ventricle fails to overcome the increased pulmonary vascular resistance in order to increase pulmonary blood flow in response to exercise at the rate dictated by the level of exercise. Also, underfilling of the left ventricle, with a resultant decrease in stroke volume, along with compression of the left ventricle by the enlarged right ventricle,[6,7] might contribute to decreased

From Wasserman K (ed): *Cardiopulmonary Exercise Testing and Cardiovascular Health.* Armonk, NY: Futura Publishing Company, Inc.; © 2002.

O_2 delivery to the tissues at low work rates (WRs). In the presence of inadequate O_2 delivery, anaerobic metabolism is initiated to enhance the energy supply for sustaining exercise. As a consequence, lactic acidosis ensues. This increases CO_2 production relative to O_2 consumption due to bicarbonate dissociation as it buffers lactic acid. This, as well as the arterial acidosis, provides a further stimulus to ventilatory drive. Thus, the high ventilatory demand contributes to the dyspnea experienced by PPH patients. Eventually, the anaerobic source of ATP regeneration from anaerobic glycolysis, used to supplement the aerobic regeneration of ATP, becomes inadequate, and muscular contraction cannot be maintained, leading to muscular fatigue.

Several other mechanisms are at play contributing to the high ventilatory response to exercise in PPH patients. The pulmonary vasculopathy in this disease results in the failure of the ventilatory dead space to decrease normally with exercise because recruitment of the pulmonary vascular bed is already maximized at rest. Thus, the physiological dead space/tidal volume ratio (V_D/V_T) is increased, resulting in a low ventilatory efficiency during exercise, which leads to an increased ventilatory response that can further contribute to the symptom of dyspnea.

In addition to increased V_D/V_T, lactic acidosis, and CO_2 production, the shunting of venous blood through a patent foramen ovale in response to exercise causes an increase in functional dead space which further increases the ventilatory requirement. The reduced arterial O_2 saturation and shunted CO_2 and H^+ stimulate the carotid bodies, causing a further increase in ventilatory drive. With all of these mechanisms operative, it is understandable why dyspnea is the most frequent early symptom of patients with PPH.

In summary, the symptoms of dyspnea and fatigue in PPH can be a result of:

1. An inadequate increase in O_2 transport to tissues during exercise, which can be measured with cardiopulmonary exercise testing (CPET) as a decrease in peak $\dot{V}O_2$, decreased anaerobic threshold (AT), and decrease in aerobic response to the imposed WR ($\Delta\dot{V}O_2/\Delta WR$) compared to normal.

2. Early lactic acidosis, measured as a decrease in AT, causing increased ventilatory drive.

3. Underperfusion of ventilated lung, measured as a high $\dot{V}E/\dot{V}CO_2$ at the AT (termed "ventilatory efficiency").[8]

4. Arterial hypoxemia due to right-to-left shunting across a patent foramen ovale, driven by increased pulmonary vascular resistance (in about 30% to 40% of patients with PPH).

Measuring Disease Severity in PPH

Standard Measures of Severity

Invasive hemodynamic testing is commonly performed before and after initiation of treatment.[9] Hemodynamics, however, do not provide sufficient evidence that patients derive benefit, or lack thereof, from vasodilator therapy. Also, evaluating PPH patients with invasive hemodynamic measurements subjects them to significant morbidity and mortality risks.

In many patients with PPH, the acute hemodynamic response to vasodilators does not predict long-term hemodynamic response[10,11]; also, the long-term hemodynamic response does not appear to correlate with physiological improvements in $\dot{V}E/\dot{V}CO_2$ nor with New York Heart Association (NYHA) class. It is a common observation that some patients with very high pulmonary arterial pressures are much less ill than their counterparts with only moderately elevated pressures.

Vasodilator therapy does not necessarily derive its benefit from improved hemodynamics, but rather from ultrastructural changes in the pulmonary vasculature itself.[3,12] These changes allow blood flow to increase through the pulmonary capillary bed during exercise, therein making CPET an ideal test for quantifying ventilatory efficiency and for quantifying the overall ability to increase pulmonary blood flow during exercise.

Finally, symptoms are not always reliable indicators of disease severity, echocardiography cannot accurately measure pulmonary blood flow, and while the 6-minute walk test provides some prognostic ability for groups of patients, its use for the individual patient remains limited.

Rationale for CPET in PPH

The application of CPET for measuring severity in PPH patients with right heart failure is adapted from its application in assessing patients with left heart failure. The NYHA has recently revised its criteria to characterize patients with left heart failure to incorporate objective measurements of exercise capacity with CPET.[13] CPET measurements, including peak $\dot{V}O_2$ and AT, are now the standard for diagnosis, clinical follow-up, and prognostication[14,15] in left heart failure. In PPH the pulmonary circulatory impairment and right ventricular failure can be closely likened to the systemic circulatory impairment due to left ventricular failure. Like with left heart failure, patients with PPH become symptomatic during exercise. This is precisely what CPET measures—functional abnormalities with exercise that are far more descriptive than any resting hemodynamic or functional measurement.

CPET Protocol for PPH Patients

In our laboratory we use the following protocol to evaluate PPH patients, and have used the same protocol to reevaluate the patients after the start of treatment.

Protocol

While seated on a stationary cycle ergometer, the patient breathes through a mouthpiece with a nose clip in place. Breath-by-breath measurements of respiratory rate, $\dot{V}_E$, $\dot{V}_{O_2}$, $\dot{V}_{CO_2}$, end-tidal P_{O_2} and P_{CO_2}, O_2 pulse, and ventilatory equivalents for O_2 and CO_2 are obtained at rest for 3 minutes, followed by 3 minutes of unloaded cycling at 60 rpm, which in turn is followed by a progressively increasing WR to the point of symptom-limited exercise.

A WR of 5 to 15 W/min is chosen, based on clinical appraisal, in an attempt to prevent excessively short or long test durations. The patient exercises until becoming sufficiently symptomatic to cause him or her to stop. The duration of the exercise period is usually about 10 minutes, with the $\dot{V}_{O_2}$-limiting exercise lasting only 1 to 2 minutes. Respiratory gas exchange, ventilation, and heart rate are measured throughout rest, exercise, and early recovery. Peak exercise values are used to identify peak $\dot{V}_{O_2}$, peak O_2 pulse, and peak heart rate. In addition to peak exercise values, $\Delta\dot{V}_{O_2}/\Delta WR$, the slope of $\dot{V}_E$ vs. $\dot{V}_{CO_2}$ over the linear range, the AT (v-slope method[16]), and the $\dot{V}_E/\dot{V}_{CO_2}$ at the AT are measured from submaximal exercise data. Blood pressure and 12-lead electrocardiographic recordings are obtained at rest and during exercise for monitoring heart rate and rhythm during the test.

Safety of CPET in PPH

Because the studies are performed with a physician present, with close monitoring of symptoms, vital signs, and electrocardiogram, CPET is generally safe for PPH patients with all grades of severity. The use of cycle ergometry minimizes the variability in the $\dot{V}_{O_2}$ response to exercise. With a treadmill, the $\dot{V}_{O_2}$ response at a given speed and grade is variable from one subject to another and less precise from time to time. With the cycle, the aerobic efficiency is uniform in all subjects, and $\dot{V}_{O_2}$ increases at a constant rate of approximately 10 mL/min/W ($\Delta\dot{V}_{O_2}/\Delta WR$) with a standard deviation of ± 0.7 in normal subjects. Cycle ergometry exercise also offers an advantage over treadmill exercise because with the cycle ergometer the patient can stop cycling on his or her own volition, whereas the patient cannot stop walking on the treadmill until the technician makes the decision to turn off the treadmill. Also, there is less risk of falling from the cycle ergometer should the patient become weak and/or dizzy. Clinicians still concerned about maximal exercise testing in PPH can choose to end the test when an apparent AT is reached, which will still allow quantification of the AT, $\Delta\dot{V}_{O_2}/\Delta WR$, and $\dot{V}_E/\dot{V}_{CO_2}$.

Specific CPET Findings in PPH

Ventilatory Efficiency

CPET measures ventilatory efficiency, which reflects the degree of V/Q mismatch: $\dot{V}_E/\dot{V}_{CO_2}$ is directly influenced by the quantity of blood flowing to ventilated lung per unit time. The pulmonary vasculopathy in PPH causes a decrease in perfusion of ventilated lung, thereby increasing dead space ventilation.[6] Thus, in PPH, ventilation relative to CO_2 production is high.

In normal patients, the dead space ventilation is about one third of the breath but decreases to about one fifth of the breath with exercise.[5] Thus, $\dot{V}E/\dot{V}CO_2$ and the relative dead space decrease in the transition from rest to exercise. During exercise, $\dot{V}E/\dot{V}CO_2$ reaches a nadir and is most stable at the *AT* (Fig. 1). In our series of patients with PPH studied with CPET, $\dot{V}E/\dot{V}CO_2$ measured at the *AT* correlated well with NYHA class[17] (r=0.5, p<0.001). The resting dead space ventilation (and therefore $\dot{V}E/\dot{V}CO_2$) is higher in PPH patients than in normal subjects at rest, and fails to decrease with exercise (Fig. 1A). This is because the vasculopathy in PPH patients prevents the normal recruitment of additional pulmonary capillary bed, thereby decreasing, sometimes severely (Fig. 1B), ventilatory efficiency. In our patients the pattern of $\dot{V}E/\dot{V}CO_2$ during exercise was distinctively different from that of normal age- and sex-matched controls, and it was consistently abnormal in our patients.

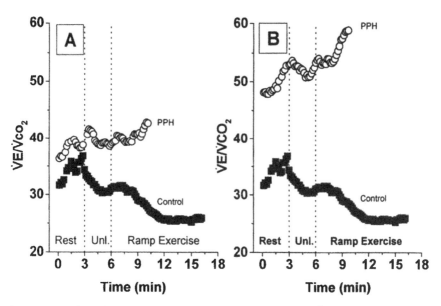

Figure 1. Cardiopulmonary exercise testing measurements of $\dot{V}O_2$ versus work rate in a patient with primary pulmonary hypertension (PPH) (**A.** open circles = moderate disease severity; **B.** open circles = a patient with severe disease) and a normal control (solid squares). Measurements were made during 3 minutes of rest, 3 minutes of unloaded pedaling, and during increasing work rate exercise to maximal tolerance. **A.** $\dot{V}E/\dot{V}CO_2$ is abnormally elevated at rest in the patient with PPH, and fails to fall with exercise, reflecting abnormal ventilation/perfusion mismatch. The additional rise during late exercise has been shown to be due to ventilatory compensation for metabolic acidosis. **B.** A patient with more clinically severe disease is compared to the same normal control subject. In the PPH patient, resting $\dot{V}E/\dot{V}CO_2$ is further elevated, and increases further to extremely high levels with exercise. Unl. = unloaded cycle pedaling.

Aerobic Capacity

CPET quantitates oxygen delivery to the tissues ($\dot{V}_{O_2}$). The reduction in $\dot{V}_{O_2}$ seen in PPH results from impaired pulmonary (and thus systemic) blood flow, and is often profound (Fig. 2).

$\Delta\dot{V}_{O_2}/\Delta WR$

The ratio of $\dot{V}_{O_2}$ increase to WR increase (Fig. 2), expressed in mL/min/W ($\Delta\dot{V}_{O_2}/\Delta WR$), averaged 6.3±15 in our group of PPH patients, reflecting a significant decrease in slope of $\Delta\dot{V}_{O_2}/\Delta WR$ compared to normal (10.3 mL/min/W).

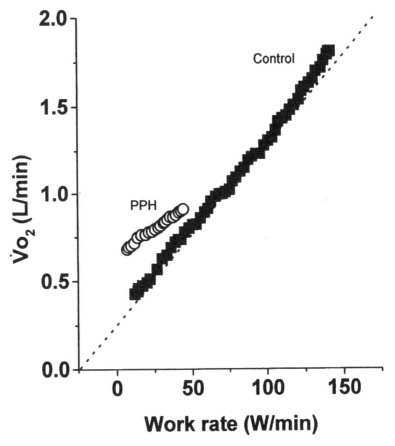

Figure 2. Cardiopulmonary exercise testing measurements of $\dot{V}_{O_2}$ versus work rate (WR) in a patient with primary pulmonary hypertension (open circles) and a normal control (solid squares). The dotted line indicates a slope of $\Delta\dot{V}_{O_2}/\Delta WR$ of 10 mL/min/W (normal). The patient's slope is greatly reduced compared to the control. Peak $\dot{V}_{O_2}$ is also severely diminished in the patient as compared to the control.

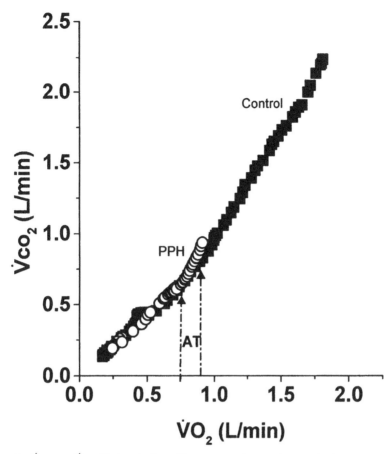

Figure 3. $\dot{V}CO_2$ vs. $\dot{V}O_2$ (V-slope) plotted for same patient and normal subject as in Fig. 2. The anaerobic threshold (*AT*) occurs much earlier in the PPH patient as compared to the normal control. Points overlie each other in normal subjects and PPH patients below the *AT*.

Anaerobic Threshold

CPET can also quantitate the $\dot{V}O_2$ at which the increase in lactate production due to anaerobic metabolism develops in PPH. In these patients, the *AT* occurs earlier than normal, because of impaired O_2 delivery to the tissues. This is seen as the point at which the $\dot{V}CO_2$ vs. $\dot{V}O_2$ slope begins to increase above 1 (V-slope method[16]), reflecting the buffering of lactic acid by bicarbonate (Fig. 3).

Other Findings in PPH

Patent Foramen Ovale

A unique CPET finding in our PPH patients is that the already elevated $\dot{V}E/\dot{V}CO_2$ is even further elevated if right-to-left shunting is present (via a patent foramen ovale). This has important clinical implications, since ventilatory equivalents appear to be an accurate marker of underperfusion of ventilated lung. If one were to evaluate CPET findings in a patient with right-to-left shunting, the reduction in ventilatory efficiency could be overestimated. However, because the gas exchange reflecting a right-to-left shunt in patients with patent foramen ovale can easily be measured using CPET, a high $\dot{V}_E/\dot{V}_{CO_2}$ resulting from this problem is relatively easily recognized.[18]

Correlation of CPET with Traditional Severity Indicators

In our series of patients with PPH who underwent CPET at baseline, a significant correlation of peak $\dot{V}_{O_2}$ with NYHA class and $\dot{V}_E/\dot{V}_{CO_2}$ at the *AT* was seen (p<0.0001 for both).[17] However, no correlation of any CPET parameter with these patients' resting hemodynamic parameters was seen. Also, the resting hemodynamic parameters did not correlate with NYHA class. Thus, it is likely that measurements of resting hemodynamics and NYHA class are less optimal PPH severity indicators than are CPET measurements, in parallel with observations seen in patients with left heart failure.

Clinical Application of CPET in PPH

CPET is useful for assessing the severity of the increase in pulmonary vascular resistance and compensatory right ventricular hypertrophy seen in both primary and secondary forms of precapillary pulmonary arterial hypertension. CPET is likely to be as useful in PPH as it has been in chronic heart failure patients for prognosticating survival.[8,19,20] It might also serve as a guide for determining patient priority for lung transplantation; however, this application of CPET must be validated.

The application of CPET in quantifying the dosage and efficacy of drug therapy in PPH patients,[21-24] as shown in Figure 4, also needs additional study. Such information will become evident with the more routine use of CPET in evaluating patients with PPH.

Conclusion

CPET will likely be a valuable guide to therapeutic decision making in caring for patients with PPH. The use of CPET to evaluate cardiovascular performance in patients with PPH has advantages over many other techniques in that it is quantitative, noninvasive, reproducible, and repeatable for the purposes of studying the clinical course and effectiveness of therapy in PPH. Moreover, CPET evaluates the state in which patients with PPH

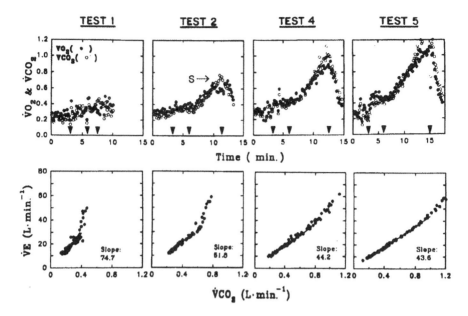

Figure 4. Four cardiopulmonary exercise testing studies performed over 12 months in a 35-year-old patient with primary pulmonary hypertension. Test 1 is prior to initiation of prostacyclin, while the subsequent studies are performed on progressively increasing doses of prostacyclin. The first row demonstrates dramatic improvements in exercise capacity (as shown by the increase in maximum $\dot{V}O_2$ from 0.35 to nearly 1.2 L/min) on therapy. The second row demonstrates the $\dot{V}E$ as a function of $\dot{V}CO_2$. With therapy, the $\dot{V}E$ vs. $\dot{V}CO_2$ slope decreases (improved ventilatory efficiency). On the most recent test, however, this ratio remains greater than normal (>25). This figure also shows evidence of shunting of blood (presumably through a patent foramen ovale) at peak exercise on Test 2 (marked with an S) which disappears on further therapy.

develop symptoms, i.e., during exercise. Also, by quantifying physiological decline or improvement in response to vasodilator therapy, it might help to objectively prioritize PPH patients for lung transplantation.

Summary

CPET can be used as a tool for differentiating between cardiac and respiratory causes of dyspnea, and when symptoms are due to both organ systems, such as in PPH. Finding abnormalities that affect gas exchange at the lungs consistent with pulmonary vascular occlusive disease and abnormal gas exchange in the tissues due to reduced tissue blood flow can be of great importance for establishing a diagnosis of pulmonary vasculopathy and for excluding other etiologies of pulmonary hypertension.

References

1. Rubin LJ. Primary pulmonary hypertension. N Engl J Med 1997;336:111-117.

2. Rich S, Rubin L, Walker AM, Schneeweiss S, Abenhaim L. Anorexigens and pulmonary hypertension in the United States: results from the surveillance of North American pulmonary hypertension. Chest 2000;117:870-874.

3. Rich S, Dantzker DR, Ayres SM, et al. Primary pulmonary hypertension: a national prospective study. Ann Intern Med 1987;107:216-223.

4. Rich S (ed): Executive Summary from the World Symposium on Primary Pulmonary Hypertension 1998. Evian, France: September 6-10, 1998.

5. Wasserman K, Hansen JE, Sue DY, Casaburi R, Whipp BJ. Pathophysiology of disorders limiting exercise. In: Principles of Exercise Testing and Interpretation. 3rd ed. Philadelphia: Lippincott Williams & Wilkins; 1999:102-103.

6. Ricciardi MJ, Bossone E, Bach DS, Armstrong WF, Rubenfire M. Echocardiographic predictors of an adverse response to a nifedipine trial in primary pulmonary hypertension: diminished left ventricular size and leftward ventricular septal bowing. Chest 1999;116:1218-1223.

7. Hinderliter AL, Willis PW IV, Barst RJ, et al. Effects of long-term infusion of prostacyclin (epoprostenol) on echocardiographic measures of right ventricular structure and function in primary pulmonary hypertension. Circulation 1997;95:1479-1486.

8. Kleber FX, Vietzke G, Wernecke KD, et al. Impairment of ventilatory efficiency in heart failure: prognostic impact. Circulation 2000;101:2803-2809.

9. Robbins IM, Christman BW, Newman JH, Matlock R, Loyd JE. A survey of diagnostic practices and the use of epoprostenol in patients with primary pulmonary hypertension. Chest 1998;114:1269-1275.

10. Shapiro SM, Oudiz RJ, Cao T, et al. Primary pulmonary hypertension: improved long-term effects and survival with continuous intravenous epoprostenol infusion. J Am Coll Cardiol 1997;30:343-349.

11. Raffy O, Azarian R, Brenot F, et al. Clinical significance of the pulmonary vasodilator response during short-term infusion of prostacyclin in primary pulmonary hypertension. Circulation 1996;93:484-488.

12. McLaughlin VV, Genthner DE, Panella MM, Rich S. Reduction in pulmonary vascular resistance with long-term epoprostenol (prostacyclin) therapy in primary pulmonary hypertension. N Engl J Med 1998;338:273-277.

13. The Criteria Committee of the New York Heart Association. 1994 revision to classification of functional class and objective assessment of patients with disease of the heart. Circulation 1994;92:644-645.

14. Stevenson LW, Steimle AE, Fonarow G, et al. Improvement in exercise capacity of candidates awaiting heart transplantation. J Am Coll Cardiol 1995;25:163-170.

15. Stevenson LW. Selection and management of candidates for heart transplantation. Curr Opin Cardiol 1996;11:166-173.

16. Beaver WL, Wasserman K, Whipp BJ. A new method for detecting anaerobic threshold by gas exchange. J Appl Physiol 1986;60:2020-2027.

17. Sun X-G, Hansen JE, Oudiz RJ, Wasserman K. Exercise pathophysiology in patients with primary pulmonary hypertension. Circulation 2001;104:429-435.

18. Sun X-G, Hansen JE, Oudiz RJ, Wasserman K. Gas exchange detection of a right to left shunt in primary pulmonary hypertension (PPH) during exercise. Am J Respir Crit Care Med 2001;163:A268.

19. Fleg JL, Pina IL, Balady GJ, et al. Assessment of functional capacity in clinical and research applications: an advisory from the committee on exercise, rehabilitation, and prevention, council on clinical cardiology, American Heart Association. Circulation 2000;102:1591-1597.

20. Stevenson LW. Role of exercise testing in the evaluation of candidates for cardiac transplantation. In: Wasserman K (ed): Exercise Gas Exchange in Heart Disease. Armonk, NY: Futura Publishing Co.; 1996:271-286.

21. Wax D, Garofano R, Barst RJ. Effects of long-term infusion of prostacyclin on exercise performance in patients with primary pulmonary hypertension. Chest 1999;116:914-920.

22. Hasuda T, Satoh T, Shimouchi A, et al. Improvement in exercise capacity with nitric oxide inhalation in patients with precapillary pulmonary hypertension. Circulation 2000;101:2066-2070.

23. Wensel R, Opitz CF, Ewert R, Bruch L, Kleber FX. Effects of iloprost inhalation on exercise capacity and ventilatory efficiency in patients with primary pulmonary hypertension. Circulation 2000;101:2388-2392.

24. Wasserman K, Oudiz RJ. Overdosing of epoprostenol in patients with PPH. J Am Coll Cardiol 2000;35:1995-1996.

15

Exercise Gas Exchange in Peripheral Arterial Disease

Timothy A. Bauer, MS and William R. Hiatt, MD

Atherosclerotic arterial occlusions in the lower extremity of patients with peripheral arterial disease (PAD) alter the hemodynamic state of the limb. At rest, blood flow distal to the site of occlusion is typically near normal in the claudicant. In response to a stress such as exercise, where an increase in blood flow is necessitated, these occlusions restrict the blood flow response. By this mechanism, blood flow supplying the limb becomes insufficient to support the continued metabolic demand of the exercising tissue, and the exercising muscle becomes ischemic.[1] Ultimately, the resulting tissue ischemia causes muscle contractile dysfunction, the symptoms of claudication pain, and the limitation of functional exercise performance.

The pathophysiology of PAD is complex and extends beyond a simple reduction in peripheral blood flow capacity. Secondary to the reduced blood flow of the affected tissue are alterations in the metabolic state of the muscle. Increased expression of mitochondrial enzymes have been identified in patients with PAD compared to controls.[2,3] As similar changes are observed in healthy subjects in response to training, ischemia, and hypoxia, these alterations appear to be reflective of an adaptive response to the ischemic state.[4-6] In contrast to an adaptation, other alterations in the affected skeletal muscle of PAD patients reflect a metabolic disturbance. Notably, the accumulation of metabolic intermediates, impairment of electron transport chain activities, denervation of muscle fibers, generation of oxygen free radicals, and acquired mitochondrial DNA damage have been previously described in patients with PAD.[7-11] Importantly, there is an association between the metabolic status of the affected tissue and exercise capacity.[8] This is in contrast to the poor correlates of hemodynamic measures and patients' func-

From Wasserman K (ed): *Cardiopulmonary Exercise Testing and Cardiovascular Health.* Armonk, NY: Futura Publishing Company, Inc.; © 2002.

tional exercise performance.[8,12,13] In light of the apparent relationship between metabolic features and exercise capacity, the relevance of integrative cardiopulmonary exercise testing in evaluating the observed exercise limitation and the pathophysiology of PAD is indicated.

In normal healthy individuals, oxygen uptake ($\dot{V}O_2$) kinetics in response to moderate, constant load exercise is considered to reflect primarily the time course of oxygen consumption and the aerobic resynthesis rate of high-energy phosphate (~P) in working muscle.[14-16] The matching of $\dot{V}O_2$ kinetics measured at the mouth to muscle $\dot{V}O_2$, suggest that intracellular processes involving the oxidative machinery (oxidative enzyme capacities) for resynthesis of ~P may potentially limit the $\dot{V}O_2$ kinetic response. Improvements in $\dot{V}O_2$ kinetics following training, with concomitant increases in oxidative metabolic capacity, support this concept of a peripheral metabolic limitation in normals.[17,18] Based on these concepts, careful investigation of the controlling mechanisms affecting the limited exercise responses in aging and disease can be studied.

Preliminary investigation of the $\dot{V}O_2$ kinetic response in PAD revealed a slowing of the time constant of O_2 uptake (τ_1) during walking exercise in PAD patients compared to controls.[19] Eight bilateral and 7 unilateral PAD patients were compared to 16 age-matched healthy controls (7 smokers). Patients with unilateral and bilateral PAD achieved the same absolute $\dot{V}O_2$ during submaximal treadmill exercise. The time constants of the $\dot{V}O_2$ kinetic response, however, were nearly doubled for the patients with PAD (Fig. 1). In addition, the $\dot{V}O_2$ kinetic response did not correlate significantly with hemodynamic severity (measured by ankle brachial index) or to the presence of disease in one or both legs (unilateral vs. bilateral disease). Thus, preliminary evidence indicates that the $\dot{V}O_2$ kinetic response is slowed in PAD, and suggests that factors other than restricted peripheral blood flow may be responsible for the apparent delay in $\dot{V}O_2$ kinetics.

There are several mechanisms in PAD that may contribute to the attenuation of the $\dot{V}O_2$ kinetic response. Other than central or peripheral hemodynamic factors, these include the accumulated metabolic changes in the affected tissue of patients that may alter the capacity for oxygen use. Specifically, the affected skeletal muscle of patients with PAD reveals an accumulation of muscle acylcarnitine, a marker of metabolic dysfunction that inversely correlates with functional exercise performance.[8,20] Consistent with the concept of metabolic dysfunction, bioenergetic data from ^{31}P magnetic resonance spectroscopy studies in PAD indicate that the control of mitochondrial respiration in recovery from exercise is altered similarly to that in patients with a mitochondrial myopathy.[21] These metabolic alterations may result from specific electron transport chain component defects and DNA (mtDNA) mutations observed in the affected muscle mitochondria of these patients.[7,9] The combination of these metabolic abnormalities may partially account for a PAD-induced mitochondrial myopathy and reduced PAD exercise capacity.

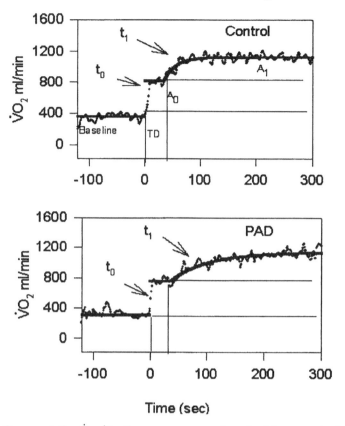

Figure 1. Representative $\dot{V}O_2$ kinetic response curves for a healthy control subject (top) and a patient with bilateral peripheral arterial disease (bottom) during 2.0 mph, 4.0% grade treadmill exercise. Exercise transitions were made from rest to exercise. t_0 = phase 1 $\dot{V}O_2$ response; t_1 = phase 2 $\dot{V}O_2$ response. Note slowed phase 2 $\dot{V}O_2$ kinetic response in the patient with peripheral arterial disease compared to control subject.

Summary

Preliminary evidence indicates that the $\dot{V}O_2$ kinetic response is slowed in PAD and suggests that factors other than restricted peripheral blood flow may be responsible for the apparent delay in $\dot{V}O_2$ kinetics.

References

1. Bylund-Fellenius AC, Walker PM, Elander A, Schersten T. Peripheral vascular disease. Am Rev Respir Dis 1984;129:S65-S67.
2. Henriksson J, Nygaard E, Andersson J, Eklof B. Enzyme activities, fibre types and capillarization in calf muscles of patients with intermittent claudication. Scand J Clin Lab Invest 1980;40:361-369.
3. Jansson E, Johansson J, Sylven C, Kaijser L. Calf muscle adaptation in intermittent claudication. Side-differences in muscle metabolic characteristics in patients with unilateral arterial disease. Clin Physiol 1988;8:17-29.

4. Elander A, Idstrom JP, Schersten T, Bylund-Fellenius AC. Metabolic adaptation to reduced muscle blood flow. I. Enzyme and metabolite alterations. Am J Physiol 1985;249:E63-E69.

5. Harris K, Walker PM, Mickle DA, et al. Metabolic response of skeletal muscle to ischemia. Am J Physiol 1986;250:H213-H220.

6. Lundgren F, Bennegard K, Elander A, Lundholm K, Schersten T, Bylund-Fellenius AC. Substrate exchange in human limb muscle during exercise at reduced blood flow. Am J Physiol 1988;255:H1156-H1164.

7. Bhat HK, Hiatt WR, Hoppel CL, Brass EP. Skeletal muscle mitochondrial DNA injury in patients with unilateral peripheral arterial disease. Circulation 1999;99:807-812.

8. Hiatt WR, Wolfel EE, Regensteiner JG, Brass EP. Skeletal muscle carnitine metabolism in patients with unilateral peripheral arterial disease. J Appl Physiol 1992;73:346-353.

9. Brass EP, Hiatt WR, Gardner AW, Hoppel CL. Decreased NADH dehydrogenase and ubiquinol-cytochrome c oxidoreductase in peripheral arterial disease. Am J Physiol 2001;280:H603-H609.

10. Lau CS, Scott N, Shaw JW, Belch JJ. Increased activity of oxygen free radicals during reperfusion in patients with peripheral arterial disease undergoing percutaneous peripheral artery balloon angioplasty. Int Angiol 1991;10:244-246.

11. Regensteiner JG, Wolfel EE, Brass EP, et al. Chronic changes in skeletal muscle histology and function in peripheral arterial disease. Circulation 1993;87:413-421.

12. Gardner AW, Skinner JS, Cantwell BW, Smith LK. Prediction of claudication pain from clinical measurements obtained at rest. Med Sci Sports Exerc 1992;24:163-170.

13. Johnson EC, Voyles WF, Atterbom HA, Pathak D, Sutton MF, Greene ER. Effects of exercise training on common femoral artery blood flow in patients with intermittent claudication. Circulation 1989;80:III59-III72.

14. Barstow TJ, Buchthal S, Zanconato S, Cooper DM. Muscle energetics and pulmonary oxygen uptake kinetics during moderate exercise. J Appl Physiol 1994;77:1742-1749.

15. Grassi B, Poole DC, Richardson RS, Knight DR, Erickson BK, Wagner PD. Muscle O_2 uptake kinetics in humans: implications for metabolic control. J Appl Physiol 1996;80:988-998.

16. McCreary CR, Chilibeck PD, Marsh GD, Paterson DH, Cunningham DA, Thompson RT. Kinetics of pulmonary oxygen uptake and muscle phosphates during moderate-intensity calf exercise. J Appl Physiol 1996;81:1331-1338.

17. Babcock MA, Paterson DH, Cunningham DA. Effects of aerobic endurance training on gas exchange kinetics of older men. Med Sci Sports Exerc 1994;26:447-452.

18. Phillips SM, Green HJ, MacDonald MJ, Hughson RL. Progressive effect of endurance training on VO_2 kinetics at the onset of submaximal exercise. J Appl Physiol 1995;79:1914-1920.

19. Bauer TA, Regensteiner JG, Brass EP, Hiatt WR. Oxygen uptake kinetics during exercise are slowed in patients with peripheral arterial disease. J Appl Physiol 1999;87:809-816.

20. Hiatt WR, Regensteiner JG, Wolfel EE, Carry MR, Brass EP. Effect of exercise training on skeletal muscle histology and metabolism in peripheral arterial disease. J Appl Physiol 1996;81:780-788.

21. Kemp GJ, Taylor DJ, Thompson CH, et al. Quantitative analysis by 31P magnetic resonance spectroscopy of abnormal mitochondrial oxidation in skeletal muscle during recovery from exercise. NMR Biomed 1993;6:302-310.

Section 4

Sequential Changes in Exercise Gas Exchange to Assess Clinical Course and Therapy

16

Changing Assessment of Exercise Capacity in Potential Candidates for Cardiac Transplantation

Lynne Warner Stevenson, MD

Evolving Separation of Function from Risk

The indications for heart transplantation have traditionally included an unacceptable level of clinical function combined with an unacceptable risk of death from otherwise refractory heart disease. Objective parameters were dominated by the need to predict risk of death.[1] Since the establishment of these indications, new therapeutic options and long waiting lists have influenced the criteria of listing for transplantation and for reevaluation of waiting candidates (Table 1).

The risks for potential transplant candidates have most commonly been sudden death or terminal organ failure from irreversible hemodynamic compensation.[2] The widening application of new technologies has changed the relative importance of these risks. Implantable cardioverter defibrillators are now in place in 15% to 20% of patients at the time of referral for transplantation.[2] Prospective data on patients listed for transplantation indicate that those with implantable defibrillators in place in fact had 2-year survival similar to that in those after cardiac transplantation, with significantly lower risk of sudden death than patients without defibrillators. This recognition has led to more frequent placement of implantable defibrillators in transplant candidates, with the assumption of lower mortality while they wait. Furthermore, patients whose functional capacity is good despite severely reduced systolic function may be considered for implantable defibrillator placement to allow postpone-

From Wasserman K (ed): *Cardiopulmonary Exercise Testing and Cardiovascular Health.* Armonk, NY: Futura Publishing Company, Inc.; © 2002.

_____ Table 1 _____

Cardiac Transplantation: Current Indications

"Absolute" Indications	"Relative" Indications
• (Cardiogenic shock) • Documented dependence on intravenous inotropic support • Peak $\dot{V}O_2$ ≤10 mL/kg/min with achievement of anaerobic metabolism • Severe refractory ischemia • Severe refractory arrhythmias	Functional capacity: • **Peak $\dot{V}O_2$ 11–15 mL/kg/min or <55% predicted** • **AND major functional limitation of patient's daily activities** • Recurrent unstable ischemia • Recurrent instability of fluid balance/renal function

Required Reevaluation:
1. **Patients informed at listing that eligibility may change**
2. **Reassessment at 3 to 6 months to reestablish indication**

ment of listing for transplantation. These patients previously might have been listed to decrease the chance of premature sudden death.

The other incentive to list patients before severe functional limitation has been concern that they will suffer rapid hemodynamic deterioration such that fatal organ dysfunction will develop prior to identification of an appropriate donor, once listed. This risk has been decreased, although not eliminated, by the increasingly successful application of mechanical cardiac support devices as bridges to transplantation. Such devices are now in place for 15% to 20% of patients who undergo cardiac transplantation.[3] The availability of these devices also decreases the concern about potential rapid hemodynamic deterioration in patients who have a good functional status at the time of consideration for transplantation.

While the early parameters of severity of heart failure often combined current clinical status and future risk of death, more recent therapies have emphasized the potential discordance between functional limitations and mortality for an advanced population. This is most obvious for the beta-adrenergic blocking agents, which have resulted in 25% to 35% improvement in survival and 8% to 12% improvement in ejection fraction, without major impact on quality of life or exercise capacity.[4] Even for angiotensin-converting enzyme inhibitors, however, the benefits for ventricular function and survival are more apparent than for functional capacity.[5] The impact of these therapies on exercise may be more to prevent a decrease in current capacity than to actually improve it from baseline.

Exercise Capacity to Assess Risk in Advanced Heart Failure

When used to assess risk of future events such as death or need for urgent transplantation, peak O_2 uptake (peak $\dot{V}O_2$) remains most useful to identify the patients with heart failure at highest and lowest risk.[6-8] Patients with peak $\dot{V}O_2$ of 16 to 18 mL/kg/min are at very low risk of imminent death or urgent transplantation in all series, with 2-year survival greater than 80%. These patients in general have New York Heart Association (NYHA) Class II functional capacity,[9] which itself is associated with approximately 5% to 10% annual mortality in clinical trials.

The threshold below which risk for imminent events becomes very high varies between studies, usually listed between 10 and 14 mL/kg/min. In most experiences, however, there is a clear division of risk at the peak $\dot{V}O_2$ level of 10 mL/kg/min, as shown in the original landmark work by Mancini et al.[6] Patients in this range have 1-year mortality between 30% and 50%, depending in part on whether they are tested before or after the adjustment of medical therapies. Many of these patients have resting hemodynamic compromise, with elevated filling pressures causing NYHA Class IV symptoms, a clinical class for which 1-year mortality is also estimated to be in the range of 30% to 50%, depending on the response to intensified medical therapy. In some patients with Class III symptoms and peak $\dot{V}O_2$ ≤10 mL/kg/min, however, the limitation of exercise capacity is due less to resting hemodynamic compromise than to the inability to mount any increase in cardiac output with exercise.[10] A peak $\dot{V}O_2$ of <10 mL/kg/min indicates an inability to triple resting $\dot{V}O_2$ to a level approximately the same as that required for walking. This may reflect low cardiac output with increased extraction at rest that reduces the capacity for further increases in extraction during exercise, borderline resting cardiac output that fails to increase and in some cases with ischemia and/or valvular regurgitation may actually decrease, and markedly impaired peripheral extraction of oxygen.[11] Severe reduction in peak $\dot{V}O_2$ is often related to the severity of right ventricular dysfunction, which itself is an independent risk factor for poor outcome in heart failure.[12] (The hemodynamic factors can be compounded by decreases in oxygen carrying capacity because of chronic anemia in heart failure.) These hemodynamic conditions reflect high risk for deterioration or death, as well as the general debility that predisposes to other adverse events such as malnutrition, embolic events, and infections in chronic disease.

The significance of the hemodynamic correlates to peak $\dot{V}O_2$ is emphasized by the work of Chomsky et al.,[13] in which those patients who had peak $\dot{V}O_2$ <10 mL/kg/min but preserved cardiac output responses to exercise had a 1-year survival of 82%, compared to 38% in those with low exercise cardiac output. Similarly, those patients with peak $\dot{V}O_2$ between 11 and 20 mL/kg/min and preserved cardiac output response to exercise had a 1-year survival of 97%, compared to 81% in patients with similar peak $\dot{V}O_2$ but less cardiac output response. When analyzing differently in terms of survivors and nonsurvivors, however, Mancini et al.[14] found no difference in peak cardiac output, but higher resting and pulmonary capillary wedge pressures in nonsurvivors.

Exercise Capacity to Assess Function in Advanced Heart Failure

While the risk stratification provided by exercise testing in heart failure is valuable for populations, it may be less useful in making decisions for specific patients, in whom multiple different factors contribute to outcomes. Assessment of functional capacity, however, is of intrinsic relevance for each individual. The willingness to trade survival time for quality of life is strongly related to peak $\dot{V}O_2$ in patients with advanced heart failure, as described by Lewis et al.[15] (Fig. 1).

Peak $\dot{V}O_2$ also provides a measure with which to compare the potential functional benefit of different therapies (Table 2). Measurement of peak $\dot{V}O_2$ after cardiac transplantation reveals that functional capacity remains limited, with usual achieved peak $\dot{V}O_2$ 12 to 18 mL/kg/min, similar to that of NYHA Class II to III patients.[16] Interestingly, heart transplant recipients often perceive exercise as being less strenuous, perhaps because ventricular filling pressures are usually lower than prior to transplantation. Measurement of peak $\dot{V}O_2$ may be particularly useful when determining function with a new type of therapy, such as mechanical circulatory support devices. Average peak $\dot{V}O_2$ with these devices in ambulatory patients has been reported in the range of 14 to 16 mL/kg/min.[14,17] The encouraging exercise performance

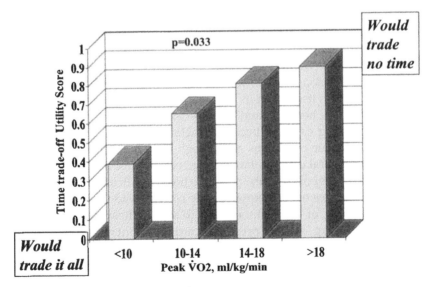

Figure 1. Relationship between peak $\dot{V}O_2$ and patient preference for survival time versus better quality of health, measured in 99 patients with advanced heart failure. The time trade-off utility score is determined during interview by finding the time between 0 and 2 years that patients would be willing to trade in order to spend the remaining time in better health. Peak $\dot{V}O_2$ is measured during symptom-limited bicycle exercise. Data from Lewis et al.[15]

_____ **Table 2** _____

Anticipated Exercise Capacity with Heart Failure and Replacement Therapies

	Peak Oxygen Uptake mL/kg/min
New York Heart Association	
Class II heart failure	15–20
Class III heart failure	11–15
Class IV heart failure	≤10
Left ventricular assist device	14–16 (ambulatory patients)
Cardiac transplantation	14–18

associated with these devices appears to reflect not only mechanical device output, which reaches approximately 8 L/min, but also a contribution from the native hearts, as the total cardiac output is approximately 12 L/min. As these devices continue to evolve, comparative functional measurements will be very important, particularly for different device configurations such as left ventricular support devices and total artificial hearts.

Selecting Therapies Based on Exercise Capacity

Timing of Listing for Cardiac Transplantation

Based on the above considerations, indications for cardiac transplantation are as shown in Table 1. These represent the consensus of multiple professional societies.[1,18] Assessment of exercise capacity is superfluous for patients with severe resting hemodynamic compromise that requires continued intensive support in hospital or on inotropic infusions. For ambulatory patients, the absolute indications of peak $\dot{V}O_2$ ≤10 mL/kg/min reflect the severe physical limitation of these patients that should improve dramatically in the absence of comorbidities that would preclude transplantation. The level of perceived limitation varies considerably, however, for patients with peak $\dot{V}O_2$ in the intermediate range of 11 to 15 mL/kg/min. Patients with sedentary lifestyles may feel quite comfortable in this range. Relentless endurance may also allow other patients to pursue reasonably active lifestyles despite frequent anaerobic metabolism. Although transplantation is sometimes performed for severe ischemia or ventricular tachyarrhythmias refractory to all other therapies, functional capacity represents the criterion by which most patients are evaluated.

Peak $\dot{V}O_2$ can improve with therapy to improve hemodynamic status, when there is initial severe decompensation, as shown in Figure 2. Considerable improvement can also occur with exercise training in patients with less severe decompensation.[19,20] Serial evaluation of patients considered for

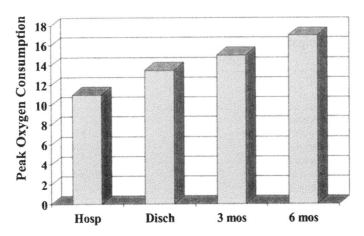

Figure 2. Progressive increase in peak $\dot{V}O_2$ (mL/min/kg) after therapy tailored to relieve congestion in patients with signs and symptoms of elevated filling pressures during hospitalization for heart failure. Therapy includes vasodilators, digoxin, and a flexible diuretic regimen adjusted according to daily weights after discharge. Peak $\dot{V}O_2$ measured during symptom-limited bicycle exercise. Data collected in 15 patients during pilot trial for study investigating impact of pulmonary artery catheterization for adjustment of therapy in advanced heart failure.

cardiac transplantation frequently reveals improvement in exercise capacity. In one experience of patients initially listed for cardiac transplantation, with peak $\dot{V}O_2$ 11±2 mL/kg/min, 35% improved by at least 2 mL/kg/min to >12 mL/kg/min and were taken off the transplant list after an average of 6 months (Fig. 3). The capacity to improve peak $\dot{V}O_2$ to this degree appeared to identify a population with good outcome without transplantation, with a 2-year survival of 85% without relisting for transplantation.[21] The value of repeated testing is less clear for populations with better initial functional capacity. In a group of patients with initial peak $\dot{V}O_2$ of 17 mL/kg/min survival was the same whether or not peak $\dot{V}O_2$ had decreased after 6 months.[22]

The approach to listing patients for cardiac transplantation has evolved.[23] Recognition of the potential for initial improvement early after referral has often led to deferral of the listing decision for several weeks in ambulatory patients. This is reflected in the past 2 years' experience at Brigham and Women's Hospital, in which only 17% of potentially eligible patients were listed for transplantation at the time of initial evaluation. Those patients initially listed had a peak $\dot{V}O_2$ of 11.2±3.5 mL/kg/min, compared to 13.5±4.6 in patients who were "acceptable" but not initially listed (E. Lewis, personal communication). The subsequent listing of those Class III patients was generally driven urgently by new events or gradually by their own increasing sense of limitation and frustration, rather than by serial changes in peak $\dot{V}O_2$. From the other end, serial testing of peak $\dot{V}O_2$ has not generally provided a reliable early warning sign of decompensation in

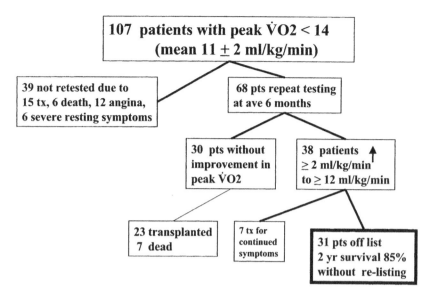

Figure 3. Outcomes of repeated exercise testing in candidates acceptable for cardiac transplantation with initial peak $\dot{V}O_2$ <14 mL/kg/min, measured during symptom-limited bicycle exercise. The majority of patients were sufficiently stable to undergo repeat testing, of whom more than half had significant improvement in peak $\dot{V}O_2$. Those with both clinical improvement and improved peak $\dot{V}O_2$ to >12 mL/kg/min were removed from the active transplant list. Their outcome at 2 years was comparable to that expected after cardiac transplantation. Data adapted from Stevenson et al.[21] pts = patients; tx = transplantation.

potential transplant candidates who are initially "too well." The Stanford group of patients with initial peak $\dot{V}O_2$ of 17 mL/kg/min were retested after an average of 8 months, and those who had declined did not have significantly different outcomes than those who remained the same.[22] The role of repeated testing in the patient who is clinically unchanged has not been established. Currently, it may be most useful in the setting of changing clinical status to confirm improvement or deterioration that would lead to joining or leaving the active waiting list.

Peak $\dot{V}O_2$ versus Other Exercise Tests

Peak $\dot{V}O_2$ can be measured easily during bicycle or treadmill exercise in ambulatory patients with heart failure. Despite their debility, even patients with advanced heart failure can perform this test safely and comfortably, with the exception of those with obvious resting hemodynamic compromise such as evidenced by resting tachypnea or systolic blood pressure less than 80, who are generally excluded. Because this test requires specialized equipment and expertise in performance and interpretation, there has been continued interest in identifying simpler exercise tests for the heart failure population.

The parameters measured during exercise testing, as for other indices of disease severity in advanced heart failure, are most distinguished at the ends of the spectrum. Peak $\dot{V}O_2$, peak watts, maximum heart rate, and ventilatory parameters all fall into parallel patterns. Patients with peak $\dot{V}O_2$ <10 and >18 are in fact usually easy to distinguish clinically without any complex measurements. The 6-minute walk distance has been proposed as an easy way to provide information on peak performance without any technology.[24] The highest and lowest 6-minute walk distances in fact do identify the highest and lowest levels of function. Across the spectrum, however, it was much less predictive of outcome than the peak $\dot{V}O_2$ in a population of 198 potential transplant candidates. Unlike the peak $\dot{V}O_2$, the 6-minute walk distance does not appear to be primarily limited or determined by anaerobic metabolism, but may be more strongly influenced by multiple noncardiovascular factors.[7] Of interest, there may be significant predictive information to be gained from ventilatory measurements at a very low level of exercise, 20 W, which is similar to that of walking (Table 3).[7] This may be important in those patients in whom peak exercise cannot be attained because of concomitant limitation from exertional tachyarrhythmias or musculoskeletal conditions.

Summary

Peak $\dot{V}O_2$ measured during exercise testing remains the most effective means of characterizing patients and populations with advanced heart failure. This facilitates selection of patients with sufficient cardiovascular limitation to warrant consideration for scarce resources such as cardiac transplantation and for major complications presented by that surgery and newer surgeries such as implantation of left ventricular assist devices. While identifying patients at high risk of death or deterioration, exercise testing may help more by providing objective assessments of functional capacity against which to make predictions of benefit from further aggressive intervention. For individual patients, serial testing may be most useful to confirm clinical suspicions of improvement or deterioration during long-term therapy for heart failure. Measurements of anaerobic threshold and peak $\dot{V}O_2$ are frequently used in heart failure patients to facilitate prescription of exercise, which can itself improve parameters of exercise performance and autonomic function. Exercise performance is a primary endpoint with profound influence on patient preferences regarding quality of life and survival. As new therapies impact patients in unanticipated ways, it is not clear how we should interpret those that may improve ventricular function without improving functional capacity. The magnitude of the heart failure population and the difficulty of selecting from multiple therapies guarantee that measurement

Table 3

Symptom-Limited Bicycle Exercise (n=307) ··· **6-Min 20-W Cycle Exercise (n=255)**

Peak O$_2$ Consumption (mL/kg/min)	W	AT (O$_2$ mL/kg/min)	Max heart rate (beats/min)	$\dot{V}_E/\dot{V}_{CO_2}$ at peak	6 MW distance	RER at 6 min	$\dot{V}_E/\dot{V}_{CO_2}$ at 6 min
≤10	48±23	6±2	120±22	58±16	300±91	1.1±0.1	53±14
10-15	82±28*	10±2*	134±20*	46±11	393±87*	1.0±0.1*	44±12*
16-20	110±28*	13±2*	142±22*	40±8	428±28†	1.0±0.1	39±8†
>20	155±44*†	15±3*†	157±25†	33±8	490±103†	0.9±0.1*†	34±4†
All patients	89±42	10.5±3.5	135±24	46±14	393±104	1.0±0.1	44±12
14±5							

AT = anaerobic threshold. RER = respiratory gas exchange ratio: $\dot{V}_{CO_2}/\dot{V}_{O_2}$.
*Significantly different from next lower peak $\dot{V}_{O_2}$ group class; $p<0.05$. †Significantly different from combined groups with peak $\dot{V}_{O_2} \leq 15$ mL/kg/min; $p<0.05$. Data derived from reference 7.

of cardiopulmonary performance will continue to be important as the field advances.

References

1. Mudge GH Goldstein S, Addonizio LJ, et al. Recipient Guidelines/Prioritization for cardiac transplantation: the 24th Bethesda Conference. Am J Cardiol 1993;22:21-31.

2. Stevenson WG, Stevenson LW, Middlekauff HR, et al. Improving survival for patients with advanced heart failure: a study of 737 consecutive patients. J Am Coll Cardiol 1995;26:1417-1423.

3. Stevenson LW, Kormos RL. Mechanical cardiac support 2000: current applications and future trial design. J Am Coll Cardiol 2001;37:340-370.

4. Lechat P, Packer M, Chalon S, Cucherat M, Arab T, Boissel JP. Clinical effects of beta-adrenergic blockade in chronic heart failure: a meta-analysis of double-blind, placebo-controlled, randomized trials. Circulation 1998;98:1184-1191.

5. Cohn JN, Johnson G, Ziesche S, et al. A comparison of enalapril with hydralazine-isosorbide dinitrate in the treatment of chronic congestive heart failure [see comments]. N Engl J Med 1991;325:303-310.

6. Mancini DM, Eisen H, Kussmaul W, Mull R, Edmunds LH Jr, Wilson JR. Value of peak exercise oxygen consumption for optimal timing of cardiac transplantation in ambulatory patients with heart failure. Circulation 1991;83:778-786.

7. Lucas C, Stevenson LW, Johnson W, et al. The 6-min walk and peak oxygen consumption in advanced heart failure: aerobic capacity and survival. Am Heart J 1999;138:618-624.

8. Pina IL. Optimal candidates for heart transplantation: is 14 the magic number? J Am Coll Cardiol 1995;26:436-437.

9. Weber KT, Kinasewitz GT, Janicki JS, Fishman AP. Oxygen utilization and ventilation during exercise in patients with chronic cardiac failure. Circulation 1982;65:1213-1223.

10. Wilson JR, Rayos G, Yeoh TK, Gothard P. Dissociation between peak exercise oxygen consumption and hemodynamic dysfunction in potential heart transplant candidates. J Am Coll Cardiol 1995;26:429-435.

11. Minotti JR, Christoph I, Oka R, Weiner MW, Wells L, Massie BM. Impaired skeletal muscle function in patients with congestive heart failure. Relationship to systemic exercise performance. J Clin Invest 1991;88:2077-2082.

12. Di Salvo TG, Mathier M, Semigran MJ, Dec GW. Preserved right ventricular ejection fraction predicts exercise capacity and survival in advanced heart failure. J Am Coll Cardiol 1995;25:1143-1153.

13. Chomsky DB, Lang CC, Rayos GH, et al. Hemodynamic exercise testing. A valuable tool in the selection of cardiac transplantation candidates. Circulation 1996;94:3176-3183.

14. Mancini D, Goldsmith R, Levin H, et al. Comparison of exercise performance in patients with chronic severe heart failure versus left ventricular assist devices. Circulation 1998;98:1178-1183.

15. Lewis EF, Johnson PA, Johnson W, Collins C, Griffin L, Stevenson LW. Preferences for quality of life or survival expressed by patients with heart failure. J Heart Lung Transplant 2001;20:1016-1024.

16. Stevenson LW, Sietsema K, Tillisch JH, et al. Exercise capacity for survivors of cardiac transplantation or sustained medical therapy for stable heart failure. Circulation 1990;81:78-85.

17. Jaski BE, Lingle RJ, Kim J, et al. Comparison of functional capacity in patients with end-stage heart failure following implantation of a left ventricular assist device versus heart transplantation: results of the experience with left ventricular assist device with exercise trial. J Heart Lung Transplant 1999;18:1031-1040.

18. Miller LW. Listing criteria for cardiac transplantation: results of an American Society of Transplant Physicians-National Institutes of Health conference. Transplantation 1998;66:947-951.

19. Belardinelli R, Georgiou D, Cianci G, Purcaro A. Randomized, controlled trial of long-term moderate exercise training in chronic heart failure: effects on functional capacity, quality of life, and clinical outcome. Circulation 1999;99:1173-1182.

20. Coats AJ, Adamopoulos S, Radaelli A, et al. Controlled trial of physical training in chronic heart failure. Exercise performance, hemodynamics, ventilation, and autonomic function. Circulation 1992;85:2119-2131.

21. Stevenson LW, Steimle AE, Fonarow G, et al. Improvement in exercise capacity of candidates awaiting heart transplantation. J Am Coll Cardiol 1995;25:163-170.

22. Gullestad L, Myers J, Ross H, et al. Serial exercise testing and prognosis in selected patients considered for cardiac transplantation. Am Heart J 1998;135:221-229.

23. Rodeheffer RJ, Naftel DC, Stevenson LW, et al. Secular trends in cardiac transplant recipient and donor management in the United States, 1990 to 1994. A multi-institutional study. Cardiac Transplant Research Database Group. Circulation 1996;94:2883-2889.

24. Bittner V, Weiner DH, Yusuf S, et al. Prediction of mortality and morbidity with a 6-minute walk test in patients with left ventricular dysfunction. SOLVD Investigators. JAMA 1993;270:1702-1707.

17

Exercise Training in Heart Failure Patients

Romualdo Belardinelli, MD

Exercise intolerance, a common clinical finding in patients with heart failure, is secondary to several factors that can be variously combined and that play different roles (Table 1). In patients with chronic heart failure (CHF), not only the cardiocirculatory dysfunction but also other associated pathophysiological factors such as ventilation/perfusion mismatch, skeletal muscle atrophy, increased ergoreflex activation, and peripheral oxygen diffusion are variously combined and contribute to the functional impairment, as described in Table 1. To determine the functional capacity of heart failure patients, exercise testing with analysis of gas exchange and ventilation should be preferred to the traditional exercise tests because only the former can provide both qualitative and quantitative information on the mechanism(s) of functional limitation and also can more accurately quantify the improvement in functional capacity induced by physical training.

The demonstration that exercise is not only safe but also serves as an adjunctive tool in the management of patients with CHF represents a recent advance in cardiology.[1-5] As a matter of fact, exercise can be considered a form of cardiovascular therapy because benefits are measurable and the "dose" of exercise requested should be accurately calculated in order to obtain an effect.[6] For instance, the combination of calisthenics and 30 minutes of aerobic exercise (cycling) at 60% of peak O_2 uptake (peak $\dot{V}O_2$) measured during an incremental cardiopulmonary exercise test increases functional capacity more than aerobic exercise alone.[5] Exercising at higher intensities generally determines greater improvements in peak $\dot{V}O_2$. Although the results of published reports are encouraging, there are several points to be clarified, such as the selection of patients who would benefit most from

From Wasserman K (ed): *Cardiopulmonary Exercise Testing and Cardiovascular Health.* Armonk, NY: Futura Publishing Company, Inc.; © 2002.

_____ **Table 1** _____

Limiting Factors of Exercise Tolerance in Chronic Heart Failure

Condition	Effect
Cardiac insufficiency	$\downarrow$ Cardiac output
Anemia	$\downarrow$ O_2 transport
Thoracic deformity	$\downarrow$ Ventilation
Anxiety	$\uparrow$ Ventilation, $\uparrow$ heart rate, weakness
Obesity	$\uparrow$ Ventilation, $\downarrow$ ventilatory capacity
Peripheral artery disease	$\downarrow$ Muscle perfusion
Physical deconditioning	$\downarrow$ Cardiovascular efficiency
Lung pathophysiology	Ventilation/perfusion mismatch, $\downarrow$ ventilation capacity, $\downarrow$ pulmonary diffusing capacity

exercise training programs, the demonstration of the mechanisms of improvement in functional capacity, and the effect, if any, on the outcome. This chapter summarizes our experience in the use of cardiopulmonary exercise testing (CPET) in exercise training in heart failure.

Patient Selection

The *conditio sine qua non* to obtain benefits from exercise training is the patient's clinical stability. In all studies, patients enrolled did not have severe ventricular arrhythmias, unstable angina, and signs or symptoms indicating deterioration of heart failure in the last 3 months. Over this time, they were not hospitalized for worsening heart failure, nor did type or dosage of medications require modification. Moreover, the majority of patients were in sinus rhythm, but atrial fibrillation did not represent a contraindication to exercise training.

Age

In a recent review, the mean age of patients studied was 59 ± 14 years.[5] The average increase in peak $\dot{V}O_2$ after training was above 10% from the initial value in all ages under 70; however, above age 70 the improvement in functional capacity was lower.

Sex

There were no differences in the results of physical training between women and men of the same age and clinical picture. The ratio of females to males was 1:4.

Medications

The combination of standard medications for heart failure and exercise does not influence the response to training programs. Patients involved in exercise training receive angiotensin-converting enzyme inhibitors, nitrates, and diuretics more frequently, and cardioselective beta-blockers and antiarrhythmics less frequently.

Functional Class

More than 60% of patients were in New York Heart Association functional Class II, and 30% were in Class III. Pretraining peak $\dot{V}O_2$ was between 15 and 17 mL/kg/min and was not correlated with left ventricular ejection fraction or with the response to exercise training. This is an important issue that should be taken into consideration when patients are referred for physical training. Patients with an ejection fraction <30% can have a normal functional capacity, and they can improve their peak $\dot{V}O_2$ more than 10% or 2 to 4 mL/kg/min from the initial value.

Etiology

As was recently shown,[5] almost two thirds of heart failure patients referred for cardiac rehabilitation had ischemic heart disease, 20% idiopathic dilated cardiomyopathy, and 10% valvular heart disease. Extensive coronary artery disease with left ventricular dysfunction and CHF are now considered indications for exercise training, because potential risks of exercise training are of greater potential benefit as compared to risk.[1-5]

Methodology of Exercise Training

The results of exercise training programs are conditioned not only by patient selection but also by the choice of the program. There is agreement that aerobic exercise is preferred over isometric or eccentric exercise. The combination of an initial warm-up of calisthenics or stretching exercise and cycling on a stationary cycle ergometer is more effective in improving functional capacity than cycling alone.[5] Electrocardiographic monitoring by telemetry is indicated in patients with arrhythmias or stable angina, and it is used in all patients during the initial 2 weeks of training. Blood pressure and heart rate are measured at rest before each session, at peak exercise, and during recovery. After a warm-up phase (10 to 15 minutes), patients exercise on a stationary cycle ergometer or a treadmill or both for 30 minutes. Before and after the work phase, a short (3 to 5 minutes) loadless exercise is recommended. The intensity of the work phase is selected on the basis of

_____ Table 2 _____

Adverse Events During Supervised Exercise Training in 154 Heart Failure Patients

Events	n	%
Sporadic PVCs	21	13.6
Sporadic PSVCs	10	6.5
Atrial fibrillation	1	0.6
Hypotension	2	1.3
Ventricular fibrillation	1*	0.6

PVC = premature ventricular contraction; PSVC = premature supraventricular contraction. *A 57-year-old woman with ischemic cardiomyopathy during stepping exercise at the end of the training session.

a symptom-limited exercise test. Since peak $\dot{V}O_2$ is a more accurate indicator of work tolerance than heart rate, it is preferable to measure gas exchange during exercise and to prescribe the intensity of the exercise regimen at the heart rate corresponding to 50% to 70% of peak $\dot{V}O_2$.

There is evidence that major benefits are obtained from programs of aerobic exercise at 60% of peak $\dot{V}O_2$ three times a week for a minimum of 8 weeks. Long-term programs are more effective than short-term programs because benefits are maintained for a longer time.[7] The results of a recent randomized, controlled trial have shown that two exercise sessions per week for 1 year can provide a sustained improvement in peak $\dot{V}O_2$.[7] Supervision by a cardiologist is preferable, especially in patients with severe CHF and with psychological problems; however, unsupervised home-based programs, more popular in North Europe, are also effective.[5] The occurrence of untoward cardiac events is very low (<3%). The most common are premature contractions and post-training hypotension (Table 2). Studies are consistent in reporting high compliance to training. Supervised programs, however, have a higher compliance than home-based programs (85% to 90% vs. 75% to 85%).

Coronary Artery Adaptations

Although an improvement in functional capacity after exercise training is related mainly to peripheral adaptations,[8,9] recent studies have demonstrated myocardial and coronary vessel changes that can contribute to clinical benefits.[7,10-12] In patients with ischemic cardiomyopathy, a common finding is the coexistence of epicardial coronary artery stenoses with different amounts of necrotic, ischemic, hibernating, and normal myocardial cells. There is evidence that 1) the presence of significant coronary stenoses in one or more epicardial vessels does not prevent an increased functional capacity with training programs; 2) the identification of hibernating dysfunctional myocardium is associated with a sensitivity of 70% and a specificity of 77% for predicting an increase in peak $\dot{V}O_2$ after training[13]; and 3) exercise training can attenuate unfavorable remodeling in postinfarction patients with left ventricular dysfunction.[14] After short-term moderate exercise training, an improvement in left ventricular contractility is correlated with increases in coronary collateralization as well as thallium uptake.[10] Since no changes in the morphology and severity of epicardial stenoses have been demonstrated, the improved myocardial perfusion seems to be explained mainly by functional and/or structural adaptations of small coronary vessels. A possible explanation may be an increased endothelium-dependent relaxation of coronary arteries induced by long-term exercise.[11] This effect has been also described in peripheral arteries after short-term programs.[15] Another explanation may be an angiogenesis effect of exercise. In the presence of a significant stenosis, intermittent bouts of exercise stimulate the expression of vascular endothelial growth factor and nitric oxide genes via a hypoxia-related mechanism.[16,17] New microvessels are generated that in part organize into large collaterals and in part potentiate myocardial microcirculation. Adenosine concentration in the interstitium of the myocardium is also increased after long-term exercise and can contribute to coronary collateral and vessel growth.[18,19]

A unifying hypothesis may be that exercise training improves regional myocardial perfusion through an indirect effect of opening preexisting collaterals and a direct effect of neoformation of small vessels. The former is due to functional adaptations of major coronary arteries determining a pressure difference between stenotic and normal arteries; the latter is related to two mechanisms: one is dependent on adenosine, another may be related to growth factors. An improvement in capillary diffusion capacity is a hypothesis that should be confirmed in humans.[20] At this time, there has been direct demonstration that an improvement in flow-mediated dilation of conduit arteries can improve myocardial perfusion. This is an intriguing hypothesis that needs to be demonstrated. Moreover, the clinical significance of these adaptations requires larger studies.

The Role of CPET

An accurate evaluation of cardiovascular, respiratory, and metabolic responses to dynamic exercise is a crucial issue for patients with CHF who are going to initiate a program of exercise training. In this setting, CPET has the following uses: 1) the selection of exercise training intensity; 2) the quantitative assessment of improvement in functional capacity with exercise training; and 3) the prognostic evaluation.

Exercise Training Intensity

The intensity of exercise training programs is variable, depending on the severity of cardiovascular dysfunction, the patient's compliance, and the finality of the program (Table 3). In patients with severely depressed cardiovascular function, the choice of a low-intensity (calculated as 40% to 50% of peak $\dot{V}O_2$ measured at the initial CPET) exercise training program might be preferred for reasons that follow. It had been demonstrated that such patients have a lower compliance with exercise training programs, lower threshold for fatigue, and higher incidence of arrhythmias. A low-intensity exercise training at 40% of measured peak $\dot{V}O_2$ three times a week for 2 months can increase peak $\dot{V}O_2$ by 17% without adverse events and dropouts.[21] There is evidence that pretraining resting left ventricular ejection fraction is not predictive of the change in functional capacity after exercise training (Table 4). However, a low initial peak $\dot{V}O_2$ is generally associated with a poor response to physical training (Table 5). The results of the largest published studies are consistent with a nonspecific response to training that is unrelated to the type of exercise, the number of sessions per week, and the duration of training. This interpretation, however, is based on the results of small studies and is not a definitive conclusion.

Quantitative Assessment of Improvement in Functional Capacity

As shown in Table 3, the magnitude of the improvement in peak $\dot{V}O_2$ after various programs of exercise training was between 10% and 26%, and was clearly independent of the intensity of the training program calculated at 70% to 80% of measured peak heart rate or 60% to 70% of measured peak $\dot{V}O_2$. The absence of a dose-response relation to training may depend on several factors. Medications like beta-blockers can be responsible for a lower increase in stroke volume after training, but they may not hamper skeletal muscle adaptations. A low cardiac output response to work rate increase can distinguish between responders and nonresponders to exercise training.[22] Nonresponders can be considered those patients who fail to improve their peak $\dot{V}O_2$ by 10% from the initial value after training.[5] In a recent study, almost 50% of patients with heart failure referred for exercise training had a normal cardiac output response to exercise.[23] These patients had a delayed lactate increase in the skeletal muscle, suggesting a normal oxygen supply to working muscles. By contrast, patients with low cardiac output response to work rate increase at the pretraining CPET exhibit early lactate accumulation, low peak $\dot{V}O_2$, and no improvement in functional capacity after the training program. This is also confirmed by our results.[7] As shown in Table 5, the absolute increase in peak $\dot{V}O_2$ is significantly lower in patients with an initial peak $\dot{V}O_2$ <12 mL/kg/min than in patients with a higher pretraining peak $\dot{V}O_2$. This suggests that central factors can be an independent limitation to functional capacity and improvement in quality of life after training. A low oxygen supply as well as skeletal muscle dysfunction can play roles in the response to long-term exercise.

Table 3

Results of Randomized, Controlled Trials of Exercise Training in Chronic Heart Failure

Authors	Year	N (Exercise/Control)	Program	Duration	Results
Jetté et al.[2]	1991	18/20	Sup,H,70-80%Hrmax,6/w,Cy+Wa	1m	Peak $\dot{V}o_2$+221 mL/min,W+13*
Kostis et al.[27]	1994	7/6	NSp,H,50-60%Hrmax,3-5/w,Run	3m	Ex time +3 min*
Hambrecht et al.[9]	1995	12/10	Sup+NSp,H,70%$\dot{V}o_2$max,6/w,Cy+Wa+Run	Sup 3w,NSp 2w	Peak $\dot{V}o_2$+5.8 mL/kg/min*
Kiilavuori et al.[28]	1995	12/15	Sup,H,50-60%$\dot{V}o_2$max,3/w,Cy	Sup 3m,NSp 3m	Peak $\dot{V}o_2$+2.4,AT+1.8 mL/kg/min
Belardinelli et al.[21]	1995	36/19	Sup,H,60%$\dot{V}o_2$max,3/w,Cy	2m	$\dot{V}o_2$+2.5,AT+1.1 mL/kg/min,W+14*
Dubach et al.[29]	1997	12/13	Sup,H,80%$\dot{V}o_2$max,4/w,Cy+Wa	2m	Peak $\dot{V}o_2$+5.7 mL/kg/min,W+46*
Willenheimer et al.[30]	1998	22/27	Sup,H,80%$\dot{V}o_2$max,2-3/w,Cy	4m	Peak $\dot{V}o_2$+0.9 mL/kg/min,W+7*
Belardinelli et al.[7]	1999	50/49	Sup,H,60%$\dot{V}o_2$max,3-2/w,Cy	2m+12m	Peak $\dot{V}o_2$+4.2,AT+3.2 mL/kg/min*

AT = anaerobic threshold; Cy = cycling; Hrmax = heart rate maximum; m = months; NSp = unsupervised; Ro = rowing; Sup = supervised; w = weeks; W = watts; Wa = walking. *$P<0.05$.

_____ Table 4 _____

Improvement in Peak V̇O₂ (Post-Pre Training V̇O₂ Difference), as a Function of Pretraining Resting LVEF in 79 Patients with CHF Who Completed an Exercise Training Program of Moderate Intensity

Resting LVEF (%)	N	Initial LVEF (%)	Post-Pre Peak V̇O₂ (mL/kg/min)
<20	5	19.2±0.9	2.75±1.6
21-24	12	22.6±1.2	1.18±2.1
25-29	31	26.7±1.5	1.58±2.1
30-34	18	32.3±1.7	1.28±2.9
35-40	8	36.1±1.8	3±3.5

CHF = chronic heart failure; LVEF = left ventricular ejection fraction.
Post-pre peak V̇O₂ difference was not related to initial LVEF by multiple analysis of variance.

Left ventricular diastolic filling has been demonstrated to be a limiting factor in the response to exercise training.[24] Patients with a restrictive pattern of left ventricular diastolic filling generally fail to increase their peak V̇O₂ after training, while patients with an initial abnormal relaxation pattern (prolonged deceleration time, early-to-late filling below 1 on Doppler mitral inflow recording) are more prone to improve peak V̇O₂ above 10% from pretraining values. Post-training improvement in peak V̇O₂ is correlated with an increased early diastolic filling. A greater early diastolic filling is associated with a higher stroke volume and peak V̇O₂, because of a lower left ventricular end-diastolic pressure and a lower transmitral gradient.

Heart failure etiology does not influence the response to training. The magnitude of improvement in peak V̇O₂ after moderate exercise training is not different among patients with idiopathic dilated cardiomyopathy and secondary cardiomyopathies.[24] More than two thirds of heart failure patients

_____ Table 5 _____

Improvement in Functional Capacity, Expressed as Post-Pre V̇O₂ Difference, as a Function of Pretraining Peak V̇O₂ Functional Class in 79 Patients with CHF in Different Functional Classes who Completed an Exercise Training Program of Moderate Intensity

Functional Class by Peak V̇O₂ (mL/kg/min)	N	Initial Peak V̇O₂ (mL/kg/min)	Post-Pre Peak V̇O₂ (mL/kg/min)
<12	5	11.4±0.8	0.74±1.4*
21-13.9	12	13.7±0.9	2.1±2.6
14-15.9	31	15.4±0.8	1.5±2.1
16-17.9	18	16.6±0.7	1.2±3.5
18-20	8	19.1±0.8	2.6±1.8

*P<0.05 by multiple analysis of variance for post-pre peak V̇O₂ changes as related to the initial peak V̇O₂.

referred for exercise training have clinically stable ischemic heart disease.[5] Patients with exercise-induced myocardial ischemia documented by positive ST changes in at least two adjacent electrocardiographic leads can have a flattened $\dot{V}_{O_2}$ response, presumably due to ischemia. This "plateau" in $\dot{V}_{O_2}$ seems to result from a delayed oxygen kinetics related to an early rise in pulmonary capillary wedge pressure induced by myocardial ischemia, and to a decreased stroke volume caused by both ischemia-induced depressed contractility and increased afterload. After training, the "plateau" in $\dot{V}_{O_2}$ response generally disappears and peak $\dot{V}_{O_2}$ is higher.[25]

A post-training increase in peak $\dot{V}_{O_2}$ is generally associated with both a steeper $\dot{V}_{O_2}/W$ slope and a more shallow $\dot{V}_E$ vs. $\dot{V}_{CO_2}$ slope, indicating a greater cardiovascular and gas exchange efficiency. In those patients whose main limitation to exercise is myocardial ischemia, exercise capacity can be improved by training-induced adaptations in coronary vessels thereby improving a dysfunctional myocardium.[6]

The presence of hibernating dysfunctional myocardium implies a greater peak $\dot{V}_{O_2}$ after exercise training.[13] Patients who improve their peak $\dot{V}_{O_2}$ after training also have an improved myocardial perfusion, which may depend in part on coronary collateral growth, and in part on a higher endothelium-dependent vasomotor response of coronary vessels.[11,12,15] A greater left ventricular contractility after training is associated with a higher peak $\dot{V}_{O_2}$.

As shown in Figure 1, the improvement in peak $\dot{V}_{O_2}$ after training is strongly correlated with the improvement in quality of life (r=0.80).[7] This correlation between peak $\dot{V}_{O_2}$ and quality of life has been demonstrated in a study in which patients were exercised without receiving psychological support or diet counseling. These data have been confirmed in other studies, and suggest that physical conditioning is one of the main factors that improve the perception of well being in heart failure patients.

Prognostic Evaluation

Not only can CPET identify patients with a poor response to exercise training, it can also provide prognostic information. A low (<10 mL/kg/min) peak $\dot{V}_{O_2}$ is associated with a poor prognosis, and its predictivity is enhanced by considering the slope of $\dot{V}_E$ vs. $\dot{V}_{CO_2}$ or $\dot{V}_E/\dot{V}_{CO_2}$ at the anaerobic threshold. In a patient with low peak $\dot{V}_{O_2}$, a slope of $\dot{V}_E$ vs. $\dot{V}_{CO_2}$ >40 indicates a very poor prognosis. These patients should be referred for heart transplantation instead of a cardiac rehabilitation program.[26]

The pretraining identification of the pattern of left ventricular diastolic filling by mitral inflow velocity profile Doppler echo provides information about the outcome. A restrictive pattern implies a poor response to exercise training as well as a higher rate of cardiac events during the follow-up.[24]

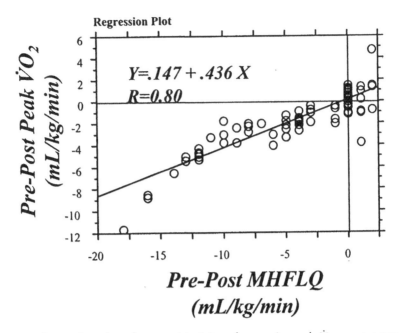

Figure 1. Regression plot of pre-post training changes in peak $\dot{V}O_2$ versus pre-post training changes in the Minnesota Heart Failure Living Questionnaire (MHFLQ) in 99 patients with chronic heart failure exercised at 60% of peak $\dot{V}O_2$ for 14 months (see reference 7).

The results of a recent trial demonstrated a lower need of hospital readmissions and an improvement in survival among patients who underwent a long-term program of supervised exercise training.[7] Trained patients, after a 4-year follow-up, had a 63% reduction in cardiac mortality and a 71% less hospital readmission rate for heart failure as compared to untrained heart failure patients. There were two independent predictors of survival: post-training thallium uptake score index and pretraining anaerobic threshold. This suggests that heart failure patients with a delayed onset of anaerobic metabolism have a better prognosis. Further, the improvement in myocardial perfusion induced by moderate long-term exercise in heart failure patients with ischemic heart disease is more important than the severity and the number of stenoses in epicardial coronary arteries, suggesting that microcirculatory adaptations are probably crucial. These results, if confirmed in larger trials tailored to demonstrate the effects of exercise training on morbidity and mortality, imply not only reduced costs but also a better quality of life for heart failure patients.

Summary

The best treatment for heart failure patients should aim to provide a better quality of life and a reduction in patient care costs. Exercise training can be considered an adjunctive tool to standard medications because it not only increases functional capacity but also improves quality of life of heart failure patients, while reducing hospital readmissions. In heart failure patients, the combination of medications, diet, and psychological counseling with exercise training seems to be a better therapeutic option than medications alone. CPET with gas exchange measurements should be preferred to electrocardiographic testing alone because it provides qualitative and quantitative information that is very useful for prescribing exercise training, for quantifying the magnitude of functional capacity improvement, and for selecting patients who might benefit the most from long-term exercise training.

References

1. Coats AJ, Adamopoulos S, Radaelli A, et al. Controlled trial of physical training in chronic heart failure: exercise performance, hemodynamics, ventilation and autonomic function. Circulation 1992;85:2119-2131.
2. Jettè M, Heller R, Landry F, Blumchen G. Randomized 4-week exercise program in patients with impaired left ventricular function. Circulation 1991;84:1561-1567.
3. Coats AJ, Adamopoulos S, Meyer TE, Conway J, Sleight P. Effects of physical training in chronic heart failure. Lancet 1990;335:63-66.
4. Kavanagh T, Myers MG, Baigrie RS, Mertens DJ, Sawyer P, Shephard RJ. Quality of life and cardiorespiratory function in chronic heart failure: effects of 12 months' aerobic training. Heart 1996;76:42-49.
5. European Heart Failure Training Group. Experience from controlled trials of physical training in chronic heart failure: protocol and patient factors in effectiveness in the improvement in exercise tolerance. Eur Heart J 1998;19:466-475.
6. Shephard RJ, Balady GJ. Exercise as cardiovascular therapy. Circulation 1999;99:963-972.
7. Belardinelli R, Georgiou D, Cianci G, Purcaro A. Randomized, controlled trial of long-term moderate exercise training in chronic heart failure. Effects on functional capacity, quality of life, and clinical outcome. Circulation 1999;99:1173-1182.
8. Sullivan MJ, Higginbotham MB, Cobb FR. Exercise training in patients with severe left ventricular dysfunction: hemodynamic and metabolic effects. Circulation 1988;78:506-515.
9. Hambrecht R, Niebauer J, Fiehn E, et al. Physical training in patients with stable chronic heart failure: effects on cardiorespiratory fitness and ultrastructural abnormalities of leg muscles. J Am Coll Cardiol 1995;25:1239-1249.
10. Belardinelli R, Georgiou D, Ginzton L, Cianci G, Purcaro A. Effects of moderate exercise training on thallium uptake and contractile response to low-dose dobutamine of dysfunctional myocardium in patients with ischemic cardiomyopathy. Circulation 1998;97:553-561.
11. Hambrecht R, Wolf A, Gielen S, et al. Effect of exercise on coronary endothelial function in patients with coronary artery disease. N Engl J Med 2000;342:454-460.
12. Laughlin MH, McAllister RM. Exercise training-induced coronary vascular adaptation. J Appl Physiol 1992;73:2209-2225.
13. Belardinelli R, Georgiou D, Purcaro A. Low dose dobutamine echocardiography predicts improvement in functional capacity after exercise training in patients

with ischemic cardiomyopathy: prognostic implication. J Am Coll Cardiol 1998;31:1027-1034.

14. Giannuzzi P, Temporelli PL, Corra U, Gattone M, Giordano A, Tavazzi L. Attenuation of unfavorable remodeling by exercise training in postinfarction patients with left ventricular dysfunction: results of the Exercise in Left Ventricular Dysfunction (ELVD) trial. Circulation 1997;96:1790-1797.

15. Hornig B, Maier V, Drexler H. Physical training improves endothelial function in patients with chronic heart failure. Circulation 1996;93:210-214.

16. Sessa WC, Pritchard K, Seyedi N, Wang J, Hintze TH. Chronic exercise in dogs increases coronary vascular nitric oxide production and endothelial cell nitric oxide synthase gene expression. Circ Res 1994;74:349-353.

17. White FC, Roth DM, Baigrie RS, et al. Exercise-induced coronary collateral development: a comparison to other models of myocardial angiogenesis. In: Schaper W, Schaper J (eds): Collateral Circulation. Norwell, MA: Kluwer Academic Publishers; 1993:261-289.

18. Ethier MF, Chander V, Dobson JG Jr. Adenosine stimulates proliferation of human endothelial cells in culture. Am J Physiol 1993;265:H131-H138.

19. Meininger CJ, Granger HJ. Mechanisms leading to adenosine-stimulated proliferation of microvascular endothelial cells. Am J Physiol 1990;258:H198-H206.

20. Laughlin HN, Tomanek RJ. Myocardial capillarity and maximal capillary diffusion capacity in exercise trained dogs. J Appl Physiol 1990;258:H198-H206.

21. Belardinelli R, Georgiou D, Scocco V, Barstow TJ, Purcaro A. Low intensity exercise training in patients with chronic heart failure. J Am Coll Cardiol 1995;26:975-982.

22. Wilson JR, Groves J, Rayos G. Circulatory status and response to cardiac rehabilitation in patients with heart failure. Circulation 1996;94:1567-1572.

23. Wilson JR, Mancini DM, Dunkman WB. Exertional fatigue due to skeletal muscle dysfunction in patients with heart failure. Circulation 1993;87:470-475.

24. Belardinelli R, Georgiou D, Cianci G, Berman N, Ginzton L, Purcaro A. Exercise training improves left ventricular diastolic filling in patients with dilated cardiomyopathy. Clinical and prognostic implications. Circulation 1995;91:2775-2784.

25. Wasserman K, Hansen JE, Sue DY, Casaburi R, Whipp BJ. Principles of Exercise Testing and Interpretation. 3rd ed. Philadelphia: Lippincott Williams & Wilkins; 1999.

26. Mancini DM, Eisen H, Kussmaul W, Mull R, Edmunds LH Jr, Wilson JR. Value of peak exercise oxygen consumption for optimal timing of cardiac transplantation in ambulatory patients with heart failure. Circulation 1991;83:778-786.

27. Kostis JB, Rosen RC, Cosgrove NM, Shindler DM, Wilson AC. Nonpharmacologic therapy improves functional and emotional status in congestive heart failure. Chest 1994;106:996-1001.

28. Kiilavuori K, Toivonen L, Naveri H, Leinonen H. Reversal of autonomic derangements by physical training in chronic heart failure assessed by heart rate variability. Eur Heart J 1995;16:490-495.

29. Dubach P, Myers J, Dziekan G, et al. Effect of exercise training on myocardial remodeling in patients with reduced left ventricular function after myocardial infarction: application of magnetic resonance imaging. Circulation 1997;95:2060-2067.

30. Willenheimer R, Erhardt L, Cline C, Rydberg E, Israelsson B. Exercise training in heart failure improves quality of life and exercise capacity. Eur Heart J 1998;19:774-781.

18

Exercise Testing to Monitor Heart Failure Treatment

Marco Guazzi, MD, PhD

Introduction

Impairment in exercise performance is a hallmark of patients with chronic heart failure (CHF) that may be documented from the initial stages of the syndrome.[1] Understanding the pathophysiology of exercise intolerance is important because it can provide basic information concerning therapy and prognosis. Accordingly, the traditional goal of CHF therapy has been to enhance exercise tolerance and to reduce symptoms in patients with functional disability.

The development of a variety of exercise testing techniques and protocols has contributed significantly to our understanding of the exercise intolerance associated with the disease. Cardiopulmonary exercise testing (CPET) is a necessary component in the acquisition of prognostic information and in the assessment of effectiveness of the therapeutic strategies. In addition, CPET, at variance with other nonmetabolic exercise evaluations, provides a means for the identification of mechanisms, other than cardiac dysfunction, that contribute to functional limitation.

In fact, some of the effects of antifailure therapies, such as improvement in functional capacity and peak exercise oxygen uptake (peak $\dot{V}O_2$), are not merely mediated by changes in cardiac performance but may involve several organ systems.[2]

CPET offers a unique opportunity for investigating the relevance of peripheral and ventilatory abnormalities in causing exercise intolerance in CHF. Additional features that make CPET an attractive tool for monitoring therapeutic benefits are the high reproducibility and its independence of the motivation of the subject and/or operator.

From Wasserman K (ed): *Cardiopulmonary Exercise Testing and Cardiovascular Health.* Armonk, NY: Futura Publishing Company, Inc.; © 2002.

Most therapeutic interventions that improve morbidity and survival generally are also reflected in peak $\dot{V}O_2$, a powerful independent predictor of outcome.[3] Improvement in peak $\dot{V}O_2$ over time is regarded as a reliable and objective index of better exercise capacity and of therapeutic effectiveness.[4]

In very recent years, however, further exercise indices and CPET-derived parameters have been identified and proposed as complementary or, in some cases, as alternative markers of exercise disability and prognosis in CHF patients.[5]

In this chapter the following questions are addressed: 1) Is CPET a suitable tool to assess and monitor the efficacy of various drug treatments in CHF?; 2) Are there consistent advantages in the use of expired gas analysis compared with other exercise testing techniques?; and 3) Is CPET of value to better understand the mechanism of action of different drugs and therefore to guide in the selection of treatment?

Monitoring Therapeutic Effectiveness: The Value of Recording Gas Exchange

Exercise performance is strictly dependent on the combined activity of several organ systems, whose integrated response allows for an augmented $\dot{V}O_2$ from air and a paired-matched O_2 extraction from the periphery. Measuring $\dot{V}O_2$ and CO_2 production ($\dot{V}CO_2$) at the mouth level provides a reliable assessment of variations in gas kinetics occurring at a cellular level. As a consequence, any improvement in $\dot{V}O_2$ reflects an improved coupling between the external and internal respiration.[6]

On this basis, exercise capacity, and more precisely peak $\dot{V}O_2$, is frequently used as an endpoint in intervention trials in patients with CHF.[4,7] An important consideration that is perhaps frequently overlooked is that the information provided by a CPET is not limited to the simple peak $\dot{V}O_2$ quantification, but includes a number of details regarding the major determinants of the improved exercise capacity and $\dot{V}O_2$ itself.

From a physiological point of view, $\dot{V}O_2$ is defined by the following equations:

$$\dot{V}O_2 = Q \times (\Delta_{a\text{-}v}O_2);$$

$$\dot{V}O_2 = \dot{V}E \times (FiO_2\text{-}FeO_2)^*$$

$$\dot{V}O_2 = D \times A/L \times (P_{cap}O_2\text{-}P_{mit}O_2)$$

Equation 1 describes the classic Fick principle (where Q = cardiac output, and $\Delta_{a\text{-}v}O_2$ = arteriovenous oxygen content difference); equation 2 describes the mutual relationship between $\dot{V}O_2$ and ventilation (where $\dot{V}E$ = effective

---

*For a given barometric pressure, air temperature, and humidity.

ventilation; FiO_2 = inspiratory oxygen fraction, and FeO_2 = expiratory oxygen fraction, corrected for the difference between expired and inspired volume); equation 3 describes oxygen transport from the systemic capillaries to the mitochondria (where D = constant describing O_2 diffusion properties for tissue from the capillary bed to the mitochondria; A = surface area for diffusion; L = mean length between capillary bed and mitochondria; $P_{cap}O_2$ = oxygen pressure in the capillary bed; $P_{mit}O_2$ = oxygen pressure in the mitochondria). According to these equations, $\dot{V}O_2$ is dependent on a complex interplay of multiple central and peripheral physiological determinants. As a final result, an improved $\dot{V}O_2$ may reflect a better O_2 delivery (i.e., isolated or combined influence on heart, lungs, systemic and pulmonary circulation, and blood) and/or a peripheral effect (i.e., improvement of impaired muscle perfusion and/or O_2 utilization).

Although a detailed discussion of $\dot{V}O_2$ determinants is beyond the scope of this chapter, it is of relevance to stress that the relative contribution of the above-mentioned factors may be comprehensively assessed by using gas exchange analysis, and the specific definition of each of them has obvious important therapeutic implications.

As reported in Table 1, the "ideal" exercise test for monitoring therapeutic effectiveness in CHF should be feasible, objective, reproducible, and predictive of clinical benefits and outcome. There is no doubt that collection of expired gases has the intrinsic limitation related to its complexity. Proficient personnel and careful metabolic cart calibrations are fundamental premises in order to obtain reliable and reproducible data. As a matter of fact, these requirements seem to be limiting factors in large clinical trials when assessing exercise capacity in studies involving a large population of patients in which repeated quality control measures are requested. Remarkably, in the VHeFT II trial, among 4983 CPET tests completed, 9.5% did not fulfill the quality criteria established in the protocol[8] and were withdrawn from the study. For this reason, exercise duration as a means for assessing exercise capacity has gained more popularity as an endpoint in multicenter trials. On the other hand, several points must be considered when making a head-to-head comparison between peak $\dot{V}O_2$ and simple exercise time for assessing exercise capacity in CHF (Table 2). A considerable amount of

_____ **Table 1** _____

Features of the "Ideal" Exercise Test for Monitoring Therapeutic Effectiveness in Heart Failure

- Feasible
- Objective
  - *Representative of maximal exercise performance*
  - *Unrelated to the motivation of the patient and/or the operator*
  - *Unrelated to day-to-day variability in symptoms*
- Reproducible
- Predictive of clinical benefits and outcome

_____ Table 2 _____

Head-to-Head Comparison Between CPET and Nonmetabolic Exercise Testing Evaluation in Heart Failure

	CPET (Peak $\dot{V}O_2$)	Nonmetabolic (Exercise Time)
Methodological		
Feasibility	$--$	$+++$
Reproducibility	$+++$	$+$
Patients' liking	$-/+$	$+$
Clinical		
Relationship with symptoms	$-$	$+$
Risk stratification (Selection for HTX)	$+++$	$-$
Prognostic information	$++++$	$++$
Pathophysiological		
Identification of the organ system responsible for exercise limitation	$++++$	$-/+$

CPET = cardiopulmonary exercise testing; CPX = cardiopulmonary exercise; HTX = heart transplantation.

information derived from gas exchange analysis makes the physician more confident that common problems related to the lack of objective markers of exercise performance and to the confounding effect of motivation of the patient and the investigator can be avoided.

Changes with transition from a predominantly aerobic to a combined aerobic and anaerobic metabolism result in the gas exchange anaerobic threshold, a physiological objective marker, not influenced by exercise time and symptoms,[9] that defines the level of $\dot{V}O_2$ above which lactic acidosis develops with its physiological consequences. The time constant (τ) of $\dot{V}O_2$ is another objective marker of the ability of the circulation to transport O_2 and has been found to be related to peak $\dot{V}O_2$.[10] It does not require the subject's maximal effort and can be obtained even when the anaerobic threshold has not been reached.[11]

Variations in peak $\dot{V}O_2$ and, possibly in peak exercise time, however, do not necessarily reflect changes in symptomatic status, especially because patients may have a psychological reticence to perform the test. Also, a nonlinear relation between peak $\dot{V}O_2$, symptoms, and quality of life has been shown repeatedly.[12]

The VHeFT II trial[13] was the first large-scale study to clearly demonstrate in a wide CHF population a dissociation between changes in measured quality of life score and peak $\dot{V}O_2$. Wilson and coworkers[14] have consistently reported that in patients with CHF and severe exercise limitation (peak $\dot{V}O_2$ <14 mL/kg/min) undergoing serial CPET tests, a low peak $\dot{V}O_2$ was associated, in 45% of cases, with few or no exertional symptoms.

These findings call into question the relevance of dealing with a reproducible exercise test as a function of symptoms and, particularly, as a function

_____ Table 3 _____

CPET Reliability in Detecting the Central and/or Peripheral Limitation to Exercise

Limitation	Information	Indices
Ventilatory	++++	$\dot{V}E$ vs. $\dot{V}CO_2$ slope, TV, Rf, V_D/V_T, $PETCO_2$, $PETO_2$
Cardiac	+++	HRR, $HR/\dot{V}O_2$, peak O_2 pulse, $\dot{V}O_2$ time constant (τ)
Muscular	++	$\Delta\dot{V}O_2/\Delta WR$
Energetic	+	Respiratory quotient (RER)

$\dot{V}E$ vs. $\dot{V}CO_2$ slope over range below ventilatory compensatory point = ventilation to CO_2 production; TV = tidal volume; Rf = respiratory frequency; $PETCO_2$, $PETO_2$ = end-tidal partial pressure of CO_2 and O_2; HRR = heart rate reserve; $HR/\dot{V}O_2$ ratio = heart rate to $\dot{V}O_2$; $\Delta\dot{V}O_2/\Delta WR$ = ratio of variations in the rate of O_2 uptake increase to work rate increase; CPET = cardiopulmonary exercise testing.

of the severity of the impairment in exercise capacity. Such information becomes invaluable when assessing the response to, and the efficacy of, medical therapy in CHF. The $\dot{V}O_2$ reproducibility has been reported between 4% and 6% in the control population.[15] A short-term study reports the coefficient of variation for $\dot{V}O_2$, $\dot{V}CO_2$, and $\dot{V}E$ to be between 2.7% and 5.7% in a small population of patients with severe CHF.[16] Similarly, but in a selected group of elderly CHF patients (>70 years old), Marburger et al.[17] reported that the day-to-day peak coefficient of variation for $\dot{V}O_2$ is less than 10%. According to data obtained in the long term (>3 months, average of 5 tests for each patient), the coefficient of variation for gas exchange variables remains low (<10.5%).[18]

Although exercise time per se may be reasonably predictive of prognosis, peak $\dot{V}O_2$ and overall CPET performance remain critical in risk stratification and assessment of heart transplantation priority.[19] Likewise, what probably makes CPET an invaluable investigational tool is the possibility that it can identify the organ system limiting exercise performance. Cardiovascular, ventilatory, and peripheral variables may be systematically analyzed (Table 3), so that the relative contribution of each in the overall exercise performance is defined. As exemplified in the next sections of this chapter, this approach represents a step forward in exploring the mechanisms whereby various drug treatments can be beneficial.

Vasodilator Drugs

The introduction of vasodilator therapy for patients with CHF has been an initially successful therapeutic achievement that has led to important benefits for hemodynamics and symptoms. Some pioneering studies with nitroprusside and nitrates demonstrated that drugs with pure peripheral action were able to improve hemodynamics and exercise time.[20] However, the combination therapy of hydralazine plus isosorbide-dinitrate (hydr-iso), as tested in the Veterans Administration Studies, was the first vasodilator regimen capable of reducing mortality and improving peak $\dot{V}O_2$ as well.[13] In terms of exercise capacity, the results of VHeFT I and VHeFT II were remarkable in that a CPET was used, for the first time, in a large CHF clinical trial and peak $\dot{V}O_2$ clearly emerged as one of the strongest independent predictors of mortality.[21]

Mechanisms proposed for the short- and long-term efficacy of this vasodilator combination on peak $\dot{V}O_2$ are an overall improvement in cardiac output response and peripheral blood flow distribution. The chronic "unloading" effect on the heart, mainly on the reduction of right ventricular filling pressure and pulmonary pressure, suggests that the favorable influence on cardiac output response to exercise may be mediated through a favorable ventricular chamber interaction and increased left ventricular preload reserve.[22] As illustrated in Figure 1, in VHeFT I, the amelioration of peak $\dot{V}O_2$ with the hydr-iso combination was not duplicated by the alpha-1-blocker prazosin. In the VHeFT II trial, in which patients were randomized to hydr-iso or to the angiotensin-converting enzyme (ACE) inhibitor enala-

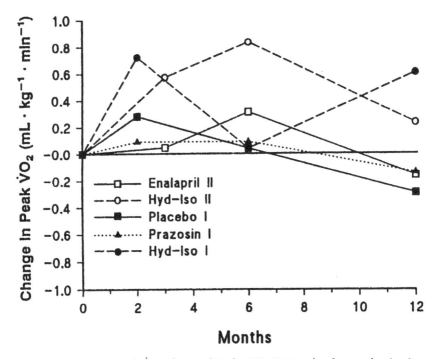

Figure 1. Changes in peak $\dot{V}O_2$ observed in the VHeFT I study after randomization to three treatments groups, placebo, prazosin and hydr-iso and in VHeFT II after randomization in two treatment groups (hydr-iso, enalapril). Reproduced from reference 13.

pril, the hydr-iso combination produced a more significant effect on peak $\dot{V}O_2$; on the contrary, minor effects on the average peak $\dot{V}O_2$ were observed in the group receiving enalapril.

A reactive neurohumoral activation, a negative inotropic effect, an impaired peripheral blood flow redistribution, and an increased ventilatory response during exercise as assessed by the $\dot{V}E/\dot{V}CO_2$ ratio are mechanisms that may explain the lack of improvement in peak $\dot{V}O_2$ after prazosin administration.[23] On the other hand, in the VHeFT II study, the somewhat surprising contrast between a better ACE-inhibitor-mediated effect on mortality and a superior efficacy of the hydr-iso combination on peak $\dot{V}O_2$ may be justified by the different mortality rate and dropouts from exercise testing in the two treatment arms.[13]

Concerning Ca^{2+} channel blockers, there is convincing evidence that the first-generation compounds administered chronically lead to significant adverse clinical events and fail to benefit $\dot{V}O_2$ and exercise performance.[24,25] Nevertheless, nonvascular-selective dihydropyridine Ca^{2+} antagonists with a slower onset of action and longer half-life elicit lower sympathetic activation and are hypothesized to better modulate vascular compliance. This produces a more efficient ventricular unloading, resulting in improved hemodynamics, symptom relief, and increased exercise tolerance.[26] In VHeFT III, however, no differences in exercise time emerged after 12 months of treatment with amlodipine versus placebo in 118 patients with left ventricular dysfunction.[27] Moreover, in a recent large multicenter trial, addition of 10 mg of amlodipine to standard therapy was not associated with significant improvement in exercise time compared to placebo.[28] Hence, the overall benefits on exercise capacity by chronic Ca^{2+} blockade remain controversial.

ACE Inhibitors

Inhibition of ACE is one of the most effective pharmacological remedies for improving exercise capacity in symptomatic CHF.[29] Interestingly enough, although these compounds have gained a cornerstone role in the treatment of CHF patients because of their multiple favorable effects on the clinical course and prognosis, they were initially approved in view of their effects on functional capacity.[30-32] In a wide meta-analysis of 35 double-blind trials involving 3411 patients receiving chronic ACE inhibition, Narang et al.[29] reported a significant improvement in patients' symptoms in 76% of the studies, with a prolongation in exercise duration in 66%. The average percentage increase in exercise time from baseline was 19% with ACE inhibitors compared to 7% with placebo.

Observed therapeutic properties seem to be class dependent and there seems to be no significant relationship with their pharmacokinetics and tissue ACE specificity[29]; no important differences seem to exist between long- and short-acting agents. ACE inhibition improves cardiac performance and reverses, at least in part, peripheral abnormalities, leading to an increase in peripheral muscle blood flow at peak exercise and an amelioration in skeletal muscle metabolism. Therefore, mechanisms underlying amelioration of functional capacity with ACE inhibitors in patients suffering from CHF has been interpreted as largely related to structural or functional improvements involving heart,[33] peripheral circulation,[31,32] or skeletal muscles.[34] The relevance of an influence on lungs and ventilatory abnormalities observed during exercise was recently investigated by our group.[7,35,36] The pathophysiological basis for exploring these issues and the potential background for hypothesizing an activity of this class of drugs on the pulmonary function of CHF patients stand on the following concepts: 1) lung microvessels are the major site of conversion of angiotensin I (AT_1) to angiotensin II; 2) ACE is highly concentrated on the luminal surface of the pulmonary vasculature[37] and its blockade reduces the exposure to angiotensin II and enhances local vasodilator prostaglandins, mainly prostacyclin (PGI_2), and NO production; 3) NO and PGI_2 production is linearly inversely related to the angiotensin II concentration, at least at the pulmonary level, and the balance of influence of these substances critically influences permeability and tone of the lung vessels.[38]

In both short-term[35] and long-term[36] prospective studies of CHF patients whose previous therapeutic regimen did not include ACE inhibition, we found that, compared to placebo, enalapril (20 mg/day) promoted a significant enhancement of the alveolar-capillary gas diffusion, as assessed by the single breath carbon monoxide technique (D_{LCO}). This was accompanied by a parallel improvement in exercise ventilation/perfusion matching, $\dot{V}_E/\dot{V}_{CO_2}$ relationship, and $\dot{V}_{O_2}$ at peak exercise and at any paired-matched exercise load. A strong correlation was identified between changes in D_{LCO} and those in peak $\dot{V}_{O_2}$, reinforcing the concept that in CHF, pulmonary derangements related to the syndrome are a specific site for the benefits of ACE inhibition.[39] The hydr-iso combination, when compared with enalapril, in spite of a similar lowering effect on capillary wedge pressure, failed to affect lung diffusion. Moreover, the finding that the improvement in exercise capacity and D_{LCO} with enalapril may be attenuated by the concomitant administration of acetylsalicylic acid supports the interpretation that overexpression of the bradykinin pathway, and specifically stimulation of PGI_2 production by ACE inhibition, may be the mediator of this effect.[40]

In symptomatic left ventricular dysfunction, initial studies showed that despite short-term hemodynamic improvement, exercise capacity changes gradually after ACE inhibition. Full benefits on peripheral systemic circulation and vascular blood flow are detectable after 3 months of therapy.[31,32] This does not seem to be true of the lesser circulation and lung function, because a significant effect on gas transfer and ventilation was observed in measurements performed after 15 days of therapy. Of note, a decrease in the $\dot{V}_E$ vs. $\dot{V}_{CO_2}$ slope has been documented after only 1 week of low-dose (5 mg/day) enalapril therapy, confirming an early benefit of ACE inhibition on the ventilatory performance.[41]

AT$_1$ Receptor Blockers

The encouraging results on mortality obtained in the ELITE-I trial[42] with the AT$_1$ receptor blocker losartan, has not been confirmed in the ELITE-II trial,[43] which showed a lower, even though not significant, mortality rate among patients receiving captopril compared to losartan. In spite of this, AT$_1$ receptor blockers possess some pharmacological properties that make them attractive, especially when combined with ACE inhibitors. In fact, the potential of AT$_1$ receptor blockers is greater than that of ACE inhibitors for blocking the angiotensin II stimulation of AT$_1$ receptors and in enhancing AT$_2$ receptor activation. On the other hand, it has been found that part of the effects of ACE inhibitors is due to an increased bradykinin-mediated availability of endothelium-dependent factors such as NO and PGI$_2$.

AT$_1$ receptor blockade with losartan in CHF patients results in hemodynamic changes similar to those with ACE inhibition, and losartan and enalapril have comparable effects on peak $\dot{V}O_2$.[7,44] Combining AT$_1$ receptor blockade with ACE inhibition is a novel therapeutic opportunity with the potential to produce additive therapeutic advantages. Its impact on exercise pathophysiology in patients with CHF has only recently been explored. Preliminary data obtained in two recent trials[45,46] documented that combination therapy was safe, well tolerated, and produced a significantly greater overall effect on peak $\dot{V}O_2$ compared to ACE inhibition alone after 3 and 6 months of therapy in one study, and after 2 months of therapy in the other (Fig. 2). When CPET variables of cardiac, ventilatory, and peripheral performance were analyzed,[46] differences between the two classes of drugs were noted regarding lung function (i.e., reduction of $\dot{V}E$ vs. $\dot{V}CO_2$ slope and VD/VT while on enalapril) and O$_2$ utilization (i.e., increased rate of $\dot{V}O_2$ per watt of work while on losartan) that were synergistic in improving peak $\dot{V}O_2$ when the two classes of drugs were combined (Fig. 3). Combination therapy also produced a greater neurohumoral deactivation whose putative role in improving exercise capacity warrants further investigation. The question concerning the role of the combination therapy and its influences on exercise performance will possibly receive further answers from by the ongoing Val-HeFT multicenter trial.[47]

Beta-Adrenergic Receptor Blockers

Long-term beta-receptor blockade improves the functional and the biological properties of the failing heart, slows the progression of the disease, and increases life expectancy.[48]

Changes in $\dot{V}O_2$ and maximal exercise performance do not seem to be factors that benefit from beta-blockers. As reported in Table 4, there is evidence in both small- and large-scale trials that no change in peak $\dot{V}O_2$ occurs after short- and long-term therapy with beta-blockers.[49-58] Few single-

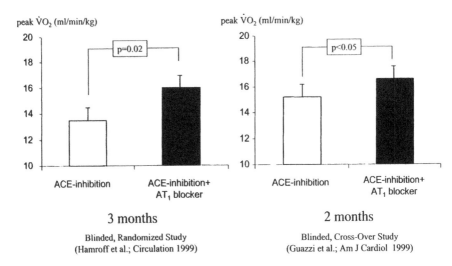

Figure 2. Evidence for a combined effect of angiotensin-converting enzyme (ACE) inhibition and angiotensin I (AT$_1$) receptor blockade combination therapy on peak $\dot{V}O_2$ in chronic heart failure (CHF) patients with severe exercise limitation. Left: improvement in peak $\dot{V}O_2$ in patients with CHF randomized in a double-blind fashion to receive placebo or AT$_1$ receptor blocker (losartan) (50 mg/day) on top of ACE inhibition (adapted from reference 45). Right: improvement in peak $\dot{V}O_2$ in patients with CHF randomized in a blind cross-over design to receive enalapril (20 mg/day) plus placebo and enalapril plus losartan (50 mg/day). Adapted from reference 46.

center studies, in contrast, have shown some increase in exercise time with both beta-1-selective[59] and nonselective beta-blocking agents.[51] In the Metoprolol in Dilated Cardiomyopathy (MDC) trial,[50] 383 patients with idiopathic cardiomyopathy were randomized to receive metoprolol or placebo and were followed up for 12 months. Compared to placebo, exercise duration slightly increased only at 12 months with metoprolol (p=0.046). This effect is possibly related to the beta-1 selectivity and to the ability of inducing beta-1-receptor upregulation. New generation beta-blockers with a nonselective activity do not induce any changes in cardiac beta-receptor density.[60] Despite a remarkable effect on left ventricular remodeling and a significant increase in stroke volume with a concomitant reduction in right atrial and pulmonary wedge pressure, their influences on exercise capacity are neutral. It is conceivable that a blunted effect on the adrenergic-driven increase in the left ventricular force-frequency relationship might limit the cardiac output increase during exercise; however, since patients with left ventricular dysfunction change heart rate more than stroke volume, the restraining effect of beta-blockade on heart rate response at peak exercise is thought to be the main reason for a lack of improvement in maximal exercise performance. This explanation may not be fully convincing for those CHF patients who do not reach their maximum predicted heart rate and in whom breathlessness and fatigue are early symptoms leading to premature exercise termination.

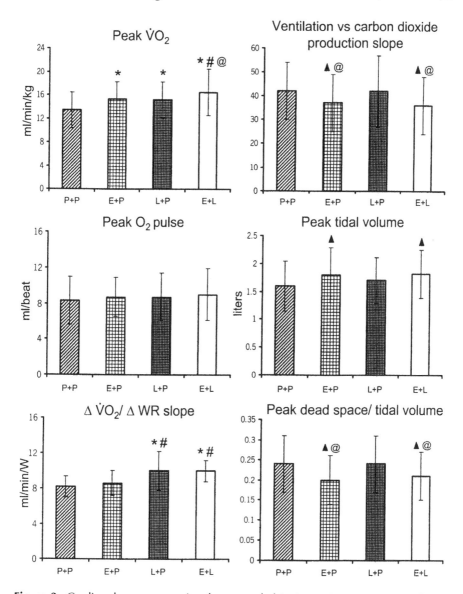

Figure 3. Cardiopulmonary exercise data recorded in 18 patients (receiving a background therapy including diuretic and digoxin) randomized according to a double-blind, cross-over study design to receive four different treatments: placebo plus placebo (P+P), enalapril (20 mg/day) plus placebo (E+P), losartan (50 mg/day) plus placebo (L+P), and the combination enalapril plus losartan (E+L). ▲p<0.05 vs. P+P; *p<0.01 vs. P+P; #p<0.05 vs. E+P; @p<0.05 vs. L+P. $\Delta \dot{V}O_2/\Delta WR$ = O_2 uptake increase per watt of work. Reproduced from reference 45.

Table 4

Effects of Beta-Blockers on Exercise Capacity in Heart Failure

Study	No. of Patients	Beta-Blocker	Submaximal Exercise	Maximal Exercise	
				Time	Peak $\dot{V}O_2$
Anderson et al.[49] (1991)	20	Bucindolol		⇔ (9.4→9.1 min)	⇔ (19.2→18.8 mL/kg/min)
MDC Trial[50] (1993)	383	Metoprolol		⇑ (76 sec)	
Metra et al.[51] (1994)	40	Carvedilol	⇑ 80% peak $\dot{V}O_2$		⇔ (15.2→16.4 mL/kg/min)
ANZ Trial[52] (1995)	415	Carvedilol	⇔ 6 min w distance (−6 mt)	⇔ (−22 sec)	
Olsen et al.[53] (1995)	60	Carvedilol	⇔ (688→871 mt)		⇔ (17.5→17.5 mL/kg/min)
Krum et al.[54] (1995)	56	Carvedilol	⇑ 6 min w distance (+53 mt)		⇔ (14.2→14.1 mL/kg/min)
MOCHA Trial[55] (1996)	345	Carvedilol	⇔ 6 min w distance ⇔ 9 min w test self-powered		
PRECISE Trial[56] (1996)	278	Carvedilol	⇑ 6 min w distance (+9 mt)		
US Carvedilol Trial[57] (1996)	366	Carvedilol	⇔ 9 min w test self-powered		
Macdonald et al.[58] (1999)	230	Carvedilol	⇑ 6 min w distance (+76 mt)		

Although a basic role of noncardiac factors such as peripheral muscular, ventilatory, and vascular abnormalities in causing exercise disability is now well established, few studies have addressed the issue of any potential interaction between peripheral abnormalities and long-term beta-blockade. Many features of submaximal exercise testing circumvent the issue of a reduced peak exercise heart rate and make it suitable for assessing changes in functional capacity with beta-blockers. According to these premises, we assessed the exercise gas kinetics and the pattern of some peripheral factors during a 50-W constant work rate submaximal exercise of 6 minutes' duration in a group of patients randomized to receive, in a double-blind manner, carvedilol or placebo for 6 months.[61] During exercise testing, data were analyzed at the third and the sixth minute of exercise, and oxygen kinetics were defined as the regression value of the slope between $\dot{V}O_2$ at minute 6 and at minute 3 ($\Delta\dot{V}O_2$ [6-3]) as suggested by Wasserman et al.[6] Respiratory rate, tidal volume, and respiratory exchange ratio ($\dot{V}CO_2/\dot{V}O_2$) were also determined at the third and sixth minute of exercise. Carvedilol, like placebo, did not produce any significant improvement in total ventilation, respiratory rate, tidal volume, ventilation to CO_2 production, and $\dot{V}CO_2/\dot{V}O_2$. The $\Delta\dot{V}O_2$ [6-3] did not vary with placebo and active therapy at 3 and 6 months (Fig. 4). Lack of an improvement in ventilatory levels and gas exchange ratio offers an additional explanation for the absence of changes in peak $\dot{V}O_2$. It

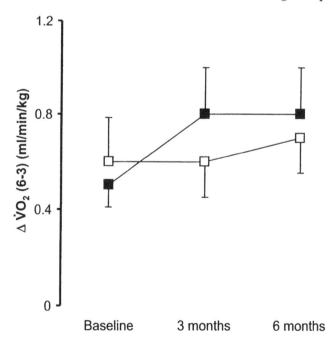

Figure 4. $\dot{V}O_2$ kinetics during submaximal 50-W constant workload at baseline and 3 and 6 months after drug randomization. Black squares = carvedilol; white squares = placebo. Reproduced from reference 61.

is also possible that the background ACE inhibitor therapy had already produced the maximal achievable respiratory improvement; however, carvedilol was similarly ineffective on gas exchange and lung function when patients were taking an ACE inhibitor.[62]

As to the effects of long-term beta-blockade on peripheral factors, sympathetic inhibition may cause metabolic changes in skeletal muscles, characterized by a 30% reduction of the fatty acid energetic source, and a greater glucose utilization with a consequent reduction in $\dot{V}O_2$ and a greater respiratory exchange ratio.[63]

Very recent evidence confirms that administration of a phosphodiesterase inhibitor, enoximone, at low doses, improves exercise performance in CHF patients, thanks to its activity on cardiac contractile state. A challenging therapeutic approach that has the potential to improve exercise capacity in beta-blocked patients will be testing phosphodiesterase inhibition and beta-blockade together in order to improve cardiac systolic performance during exercise. This should overcome the blunted increase in the cardiac force-frequency relationship caused by adrenergic inhibition.[64]

Summary

CPET in CHF allows the quantification of exercise intolerance, as well as the investigation of its pathophysiology. This has advantages over simply measuring exercise duration for estimating severity of the disease and survival and interpreting the mechanism of action of different drugs. The combination of hydr-iso dinitrate was the first pharmacological strategy effective on mortality, showing favorable and sustained effects on peak $\dot{V}O_2$.

Inhibition of the renin-angiotensin system is a most effective pharmacological approach to improve exercise capacity in symptomatic CHF. ACE inhibitors and AT_1 receptor blockers are similarly effective on exercise performance and peak $\dot{V}O_2$ and, interestingly, increasing evidence suggests that additional benefits may be obtained when the two classes of drugs are combined. Different targets and pathways are believed to be the basis for their synergistic efficacy.

Overexpression of bradykinin bioproducts and a more complete angiotensin II blockade account for a combined improvement in exercise ventilation and muscle perfusion, respectively. Beta-blocking agents significantly enhance the biological and functional properties of the heart as well as the clinical status and outcome in CHF. Remarkably, changes in peak $\dot{V}O_2$ and exercise tolerance do not seem to be part of the benefits. A reason for this might be that in most clinical trials, beta-blockers were administered on top of ACE inhibitor therapy, which could have already produced the maximal achievable benefit on exercise capacity. Alternative potential explanatory mechanisms for a lack of improvement in peak $\dot{V}O_2$ are a restraining effect on maximal heart rate, a blunted adrenergic-mediated increase in the cardiac force-frequency relation, or a lack of effect on gas exchange and ventilatory levels during exercise.

Benefits and mechanisms of action of other newly developed therapeutic options, such as antialdosterone drugs, are presently quite underinvestigated.

References

1. LeJemtel TH, Liang CS, Stewart DK, et al. Reduced peak aerobic capacity in asymptomatic left ventricular systolic dysfunction. A substudy of the studies of left ventricular dysfunction (SOLVD). SOLVD Investigators. Studies of Left Ventricular Dysfunction. Circulation 1994;90:2757-2560.

2. Clark AL, Poole-Wilson PA, Coats AJ. Exercise limitation in chronic heart failure: central role of the periphery. J Am Coll Cardiol 1996;28:1092-1102.

3. Myers J, Gullestad L. The role of exercise testing and gas exchange measurement in the prognostic assessment of patients with heart failure. Curr Opin Cardiol 1998;13:145-155.

4. Cohn JN. Exercise tolerance as a guide to therapeutic efficacy for heart failure. The potential for angiotensin receptor blockers. Circulation 1999;100:2208-2209.

5. Robbins M, Francis G, Pashkow FJ, et al. Ventilatory and heart rate responses to exercise: better predictors of heart failure mortality than peak oxygen consumption. Circulation 1999;100:2411-2417.

6. Wasserman K, Hansen JE, Sue DY, Casaburi R, Whipp BJ. Principles of Exercise Testing and Interpretation. Philadelphia: Lippincott Williams & Wilkins; 1999.

7. Guazzi M, Melzi G, Agostoni PG. Comparison of changes in respiratory function and exercise oxygen uptake with losartan versus enalapril in congestive heart failure secondary to ischemic or idiopathic dilated cardiomyopathy. Am J Cardiol 1997;80:1572-1576.

8. Cohn JN, Archibald DG, Ziesche S, et al. Effect of vasodilator therapy on mortality in chronic congestive heart failure. N Engl J Med 1986;314:1547-1552.

9. Wasserman K, Beaver BL, Whipp BJ. Gas exchange theory and the lactic acidosis (anaerobic) threshold. Circulation 1990;81:II-14-II-30.

10. DeGroote P, Millaire A, Decloux E, Nugue O, Guimier P, Ducloux G. Kinetics of oxygen consumption during and after exercise in patients with dilated cardiomyopathy. New markers of exercise intolerance with clinical implications. J Am Coll Cardiol 1996;28:168-175.

11. Koike A, Yajima T, Adachi H, et al. Evaluation of exercise capacity using submaximal exercise at a constant work rate in patients with cardiovascular disease. Circulation 1995;91:1719-1724.

12. Francis GS, Rector TS. Maximal exercise tolerance as a therapeutic end point in heart failure—are we relying on the right measure? Am J Cardiol 1994;73:304-306.

13. Ziesche S, Cobb FR, Cohn JN, Johnson G, Tristani F for the VHeFT VA Cooperatives Studies Group. Hydralazine and isosorbide dinitrate combination improves exercise tolerance in heart failure. Results from V-HeFT I and V-HeFT II. Circulation 1993;87:VI-56-VI-64.

14. Wilson JR, Hanamanthu S, Chomsky DB, Davis SF. Relationship between exertional symptoms and functional capacity in patients with heart failure. J Am Coll Cardiol 1999;33:1943-1977.

15. Jones NL. Clinical Exercise Testing. 3rd ed. Philadelphia: WB Saunders; 1988.

16. Meyer K, Westbrook S, Schwaibold M, Hajric R, Peters K, Roskamm H. Short-term reproducibility of cardiopulmonary measurements during exercise testing in patients with severe heart failure. Am Heart J 1997;134:20-26.

17. Marburger CT, Brubaker PH, Pollock WE, Morgan TM, Kitzman DW. Reproducibility of cardiopulmonary exercise testing in elderly patients with congestive heart failure. Am J Cardiol 1998;82:905-909.

18. Janicki JS, Gupta S, Ferris TS, McElroy PA. Long-term reproducibility of respiratory gas exchange measurements during exercise in patients with stable heart failure. Chest 1990;97:12-17.

19. Mancini D, LeJemtel T, Aaronson K. Peak VO(2): a simple yet enduring standard. Circulation 2000;101:1080-1082.

20. Leier CV, Huss PM, Magorien RD, Unverferth DV. Improved exercise capacity and differing arterial and venous intolerance during chronic isosorbide dinitrate therapy for congestive heart failure. Circulation 1983;67:817-822.

21. Cohn JN, Johnson GR, Shabetai R, et al. Ejection fraction, peak exercise oxygen consumption, cardiothoracic ratio, ventricular arrhythmias, and plasma norepinephrine as determinants of prognosis in heart failure. The V-HeFT VA Cooperative Studies Group. Circulation 1993;87:VI5-VI16.

22. Smith RF, Jonson G, Zieshe S, Bath G, Blankeship CK, Cohn JN. Functional capacity in heart failure. Comparison of methods for assessment and their relation to other indexes of heart failure. Circulation 1993;87:VI-88-VI-93.

23. Fink LI, Wilson JR, Ferraro N. Exercise ventilation and pulmonary artery wedge pressure in chronic stable congestive heart failure. Am J Cardiol 1986;57:249-253.

24. Elkayam U, Amin J, Mehra A, Vasquez J, Weber L, Rahimtoola SH. A prospective, randomized, double-blind, crossover study to compare the efficacy and safety of chronic nifedipine therapy with that of isosorbide dinitrate and their combination in the treatment of chronic congestive heart failure. Circulation 1990;82:1954-1961.

25. Agostoni PG, De Cesare N, Doria E, Polese A, Tamborini G, Guazzi MD. Afterload reduction: a comparison of captopril and nifedipine in dilated cardiomyopathy. Br Heart J 1986;55:391-399.

26. Packer M, Nicod P, Khanderia R, et al. Randomized, multicenter, double-blind, placebo-controlled evaluation of amlodipine in patients with mild-to-moderate heart failure. J Am Coll Cardiol 1996;(suppl A):274A. Abstract.

27. Cohn JN, Zieshe SM, Smith R, et al. Effect of calcium antagonist felodipine as supplementary vasodilator therapy in patients with chronic heart failure treated with enalapril: V-HeFT III. Circulation 1997;96:856-863.

28. Udelson JE, DeAbate CA, Berk M, et al. Effects of amlodipine on exercise tolerance, quality of life, and left ventricular function in patients with heart failure from left ventricular systolic dysfunction. Am Heart J 2000;139:503-510.

29. Narang N, Swedberg K, Cleland JFG. What is the ideal study design for evaluation of treatment for heart failure? Insight from trials assessing the effects of ACE-inhibitors on exercise capacity. Eur Heart J 1996;17:120-134.

30. Kramer BL, Massie BN, Topic N. Controlled trial of captopril in chronic heart failure: a rest and hemodynamic study. Circulation 1983;67:807-816.

31. Drexler H, Banhardt U, Meinertz T, Wollschlager H, Lehmann M, Just H. Contrasting peripheral short-term and long-term effects of converting enzyme inhibition in patients with congestive heart failure. A double-blind, placebo-controlled trial. Circulation 1989;79:491-502.

32. Mancini DM, Davis L, Wexler JP, Chadwick B, Lejemtel TH. Dependence of enhanced maximal exercise performance on increased peak skeletal muscle perfu-

sion during long-term captopril therapy in heart failure. J Am Coll Cardiol 1987;10:845-850.

33. Cohn JN. Structural basis for heart failure: ventricular remodeling and its pathophysiological inhibition. Circulation 1995;91:2504-2507.

34. Wilson IR, Ferraro N. Effect of the renin-angiotensin system on limb circulation and metabolism during exercise in patients with chronic heart failure. J Am Coll Cardiol 1985;6:556-563.

35. Guazzi M, Marenzi GC, Alimento M, Contini M, Agostoni PG. Improvement of alveolar-capillary membrane diffusing capacity with enalapril in chronic heart failure and counteracting effect of aspirin. Circulation 1997;95:1930-1936.

36. Guazzi M, Melzi G, Marenzi GC, Agostoni PG. ACE-inhibition facilitates alveolar-capillary gas transfer, and improves ventilation/perfusion coupling in patients with left ventricular dysfunction. Clin Pharmacol Ther 1999;65:319-327.

37. Pieruzzi F, Abassi ZA, Keiser HR. Expression of renin-angiotensin system components in the heart, kidneys, and lungs of rats with experimental heart failure. Circulation 1995;92:3105-3112.

38. Van Grondelle A, Whorten GS, Ellis D, et al. Altering hydrodynamic variables influences PGI2 production by isolated lungs and endothelial cells. J Appl Physiol 1984;57:388-395.

39. Guazzi M. Alveolar-capillary membrane dysfunction in chronic heart failure: pathophysiology and therapeutic implications. Clin Sci 2000;98:633-641.

40. Guazzi M, Pontone G, Agostoni PG. Aspirin worsens exercise performance and pulmonary gas exchange in heart failure patients who are taking ACE-inhibitors. Am Heart J 1999;138:254-259.

41. Kitaoka H, Takata J, Hitomi N, et al. Effect of angiotensin-converting enzyme inhibitor (enalapril or imidapril) on ventilation during exercise in patients with chronic heart failure secondary to idiopathic dilated cardiomyopathy. Am J Cardiol 2000;85:758-760.

42. Pitt B, Segal R, Martinez FA, et al. Randomised trial of losartan versus captopril in patients over 65 with heart failure. Lancet 1997;349:747-752.

43. Pitt B, Poole-Wilson PA, Segal R, et al. Effect of losartan compared with captopril on mortality in patients with symptomatic heart failure: randomised trial—the Losartan Heart Failure Survival Study ELITE II. Lancet 2000;355:1582-1587.

44. Lang RM, Elkayam U, Yellen LG, et al. Comparative effects of losartan and enalapril on exercise capacity and clinical status in patients with heart failure. J Am Coll Cardiol 1997;30:983-991.

45. Hamroff G, Katz SD, Mancini D, et al. Addition of angiotensin II receptor blockade to maximal angiotensin-converting enzyme inhibition improves exercise capacity in patients with severe congestive heart failure. Circulation 1999;99:990-992.

46. Guazzi M, Palermo P, Pontone G, Susini F, Agostoni PG. Synergistic efficacy of enalapril and losartan on exercise performance and oxygen consumption at peak exercise in congestive heart failure. Am J Cardiol 1999;84:1038-1043.

47. Cohn JN. Improving outcomes in congestive heart failure: Val-HeFT. Valsartan in Heart Failure Trial. Cardiology 1999;91(suppl 1):19-22.

48. Eichhorn EJ, Bristow MR. Medical therapy can improve the biological properties of the chronically failing heart. A new era in the treatment of heart failure. Circulation 1996;94:2285-2296.

49. Anderson JL, Gilbert EM. Long-term (2 year) beneficial effects of beta-adrenergic blockade with bucindolol in patients with idiopathic dilated cardiomyopathy. J Am Coll Cardiol 1991;17:1373-1381.

50. Waagstein F, Bristow MR, Swedberg K, et al. Beneficial effects of metoprolol in idiopathic dilated cardiomyopathy. Metoprolol in Dilated Cardiomyopathy (MDC) Trial Study Group. Lancet 1993;342:1441-1446.

51. Metra M, Nardi M, Giubbini R, Dei Cas L. Effects of short- and long-term carvedilol administration on rest and exercise hemodynamic variables, exercise capacity and clinical conditions in patients with idiopathic dilated cardiomyopathy. J Am Coll Cardiol 1994;24:1678-1687.

52. Australia/New Zealand Heart Failure Research Collaborative Group. Effects of Carvedilol, a vasodilator-beta blocker, in patients with congestive heart failure due to ischemic heart disease. Circulation 1995;92:212-218.

53. Olsen SL, Gilbert EM, Renlund DG, Taylor DO, Yanowitz FD, Bristow MR. Carvedilol improves left ventricular function and symptoms in chronic heart failure: a double-blind randomized study. J Am Coll Cardiol 1995;25:1225-1231.

54. Krum H, Sackner-Bernstein JD, Goldsmith RL, et al. Double-blind, placebo-controlled study of the long-term efficacy of carvedilol in patients with severe chronic heart failure. Circulation 1995;92:1499-1506.

55. Bristow MR, Gilbert EM, Abraham WT, et al. Carvedilol produces dose-related improvements in left ventricular function and survival in subjects with chronic heart failure. MOCHA Investigators. Circulation 1996;94:2807-2816.

56. Packer M, Colucci WS, Sackner-Bernstein JD, et al. Double-blind, placebo-controlled study of the effects of carvedilol in patients with moderate to severe heart failure. The PRECISE Trial. Prospective Randomized Evaluation of Carvedilol on Symptoms and Exercise. Circulation 1996;94:2793-2799.

57. Colucci WS, Packer M, Bristow MR, et al. Carvedilol inhibits clinical progression in patients with mild symptoms of heart failure. US Carvedilol Heart Failure Study Group. Circulation 1996;94:2800-2806.

58. Macdonald PS, Keogh AM, Aboyoun CL, Lund M, Amor R, McCaffrey DJ. Tolerability and efficacy of carvedilol in patients with New York Heart Association Class IV. J Am Coll Cardiol 1999;33:924-931.

59. Engelmeier RS, O'Connel JB, Walsh R, Rad N, Scanlon PJ, Gunnar RM. Improvement in symptoms and exercise tolerance by metoprolol in patients with dilated cardiomyopathy: a double-blind, randomized, placebo-controlled trial. Circulation 1985;75:536-546.

60. Gilbert EM, Abraham WT, Olsen S, et al. Comparative hemodynamic, left ventricular functional, and antiadrenergic effects of chronic treatment with metoprolol versus carvedilol in the failing heart. Circulation 1996;94:2817-2825.

61. Guazzi M, Agostoni PG. Monitoring gas exchange during a constant work rate exercise in patients with left ventricular dysfunction treated with carvedilol. Am J Cardiol 2000;85:660-664.

62. Guazzi M, Agostoni PG, Matturri M, Pontone G, Guazzi MD. Pulmonary function, cardiac function, and exercise capacity in a follow-up of patients with congestive heart failure treated with carvedilol. Am Heart J 1999;138:460-467.

63. Lang CC, Rayos GH, Chomsky DB, Wood AJ, Wilson JR. Effect of sympathoinhibition on exercise performance in patients with heart failure. Circulation 1997;96:238-245.

64. Lowes BD, Higginbotham M, Petrovich L, et al. Low-dose enoximone improves exercise capacity in chronic heart failure. Enoximone Study Group. J Am Coll Cardiol 2000;36:501-508.

Index

Abnormalities in exercise-derived gas exchange variables other than peak $\dot{V}O_2$ and anaerobic threshold in chronic heart failure:
blood pressure response, 85
heart rate response, 85
kinetics of recovery in $\dot{V}O_2$, 81-85
oscillatory ventilatory and gas exchange pattern, 85-86
oxygen pulse, 80-81
rebound of $\dot{V}O_2$, 85
slope of $\dot{V}O_2$/time or $\dot{V}O_2$/work rate, 79-80

Abnormalities in exercise gas exchange in primary pulmonary hypertension (PPH):
aerobic capacity findings, 184
anaerobic threshold, 185
clinical application of CPET in PPH, 186
correlation of CPET with traditional severity indicators, 186
CPET protocol for PPH patients, 181-182
$\Delta \dot{V}O_2/\Delta WR$, 184
measuring disease severity in PPH, 180-181
patent foramen ovale, 185-186
protocol, 182
rationale for CPET in PPH, 181
safety of CPET in PPH, 182
specific CPET findings in PPH, 182-185
standard measures of severity, 180-181

ventilatory efficiency findings, 182-183

ACE inhibitors, 72, 137, 138, 142, 144, 226, 227-228

American College of Cardiology (ACC):
surgery-specific risk, 122-123
transplantation guidelines, 103

American Heart Association (AHA):
surgery-specific risk, 122-123
transplantation guidelines, 103

Angiotensin-converting enzyme (ACE) inhibitors, 72, 137, 138, 142, 144, 226, 227-228

Anaerobic threshold, 23
abnormalities in exercise-derived gas exchange variables other than peak $\dot{V}O_2$ and anaerobic threshold in chronic heart failure, 79-88
and aging, 121, 131
CPET in PPH, 185
diagnosis of myocardial ischemia and cardiac failure by CPET, 124-125, 131
incidence and significance of myocardial ischemia and cardiac failure, 126-128, 131
influence of cardiopulmonary exercise on selection of patients for surgery, 128-129
in localized muscle metabolism studies in CHF patients, 29, 30, 31, 32

Printed and bound by CPI Group (UK) Ltd, Croydon, CR0 4YY

16/04/2025

14658822-0002